Contents

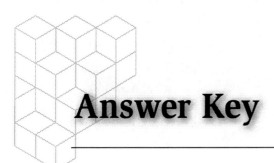
Answer Key

Question 1

Correct answer:

c. Confirmation does not require documentation of positive serology or culture for HIV.

Rationale:

ICD-10-CM Official Guidelines for Coding and Reporting 2011, p. 16, at *www.cdc.gov/nchs/data/icd9/10cmguidelines2011_FINAL.pdf*, state:

> *Code only confirmed cases of HIV infection/illness. This is an exception to the hospital inpatient guideline Section II, H. In this context, "confirmation" does not require documentation of positive serology or culture for HIV; the provider's diagnostic statement that the patient is HIV positive, or has an HIV-related illness is sufficient.*

Question 2

Correct answer:

Fifth character for laterality

Rationale:

Refer to the following note at the beginning of the *ICD-10-CM Table of Neoplasms*:

> *Codes listed with a dash -, following the code have a required 5th character for laterality. The tabular list must be reviewed for the complete code.*

Access the *ICD-10 Table of Neoplasms* at *www.cms.gov/ICD10/11b1_2011_ICD10CM_and_GEMs.asp#TopOfPage.*

Download the 2011 Code Tables and Index file.

Select icd10cm_neoplasm_2011.

Question 3

Correct answer:

b. A neoplasm code should be sequenced first, followed by a code from M84.5- for the pathological fracture.

Rationale:

ICD-10-CM Official Guidelines for Coding and Reporting 2011, p. 27, state:

> *If the focus of treatment is the neoplasm with an associated pathological fracture, the neoplasm code should be sequenced first, followed by a code from M84.5- for the pathological fracture.*

Question 4

Correct answer:

Excludes1

anemia due to antineoplastic chemotherapy (D64.81)

aplastic anemia due to antineoplastic chemotherapy (D61.1)

Rationale:

In the *2011 ICD-10-CM Tabular List of Diseases and Injuries*, this Excludes1 note appears below code D63.0.

Question 5

Correct answer:

a. E10.621 and L97.409

Rationale:

The following note appears in the *ICD-10-CM Tabular List of Diseases and Injuries*:

E10.621 Type 1 diabetes mellitus with foot ulcer

   Use additional code to identify site of ulcer (L97.4-, L97.5-)

The additional code notes include "an unspecified" heel. Code L97.409 does not specify right or left laterality: Non-pressure chronic ulcer of unspecified heel and midfoot with unspecified severity. The other codes in the range specify the right foot, as the following descriptions indicate:

L97.419	*Non-pressure chronic ulcer of right heel and midfoot with unspecified severity*
L97.511	*Non-pressure chronic ulcer of other part of right foot limited to breakdown of skin*
L97.519	*Non-pressure chronic ulcer of other part of right foot with unspecified severity*

Access the *ICD-10-CM Tabular List of Diseases and Injuries* at *www.cms.gov/ICD10/11b1_2011_ICD10CM_and_GEMs.asp#TopOfPage*.

Download the 2011 Code Tables and Index file.

Select icd10cm_Tabular.

Refer to Chapter 12, Diseases of the Skin and Subcutaneous Tissue (L00–L99).

Question 6

Correct answer:

False

Rationale:

This information does not exist in the *ICD-10-CM Tabular List of Diseases and Injuries* nor in the *ICD-10-CM Official Guidelines for Coding and Reporting 2011*. Attending physicians will need to document the severity of nonproliferative diabetic retinopathy to facilitate assignment of the most specific code.

Question 7

Correct answer:

- If both use and abuse are documented, assign only the code for abuse

- If both abuse and dependence are documented, assign only the code for dependence

- If use, abuse, and dependence are all documented, assign only the code for dependence

- If both use and dependence are documented, assign only the code for dependence

Rationale:

ICD-10-CM Official Guidelines for Coding and Reporting 2011, p. 31, state:

> *When the provider documentation refers to use, abuse and dependence of the same substance (e.g. alcohol, opioid, cannabis, etc.), only one code should be assigned to identify the pattern of use based on the following hierarchy:*
>
> - *If both use and abuse are documented, assign only the code for abuse*
>
> - *If both abuse and dependence are documented, assign only the code for dependence*
>
> - *If use, abuse and dependence are all documented, assign only the code for dependence*
>
> - *If both use and dependence are documented, assign only the code for dependence.*

Question 8

Correct answer:

Excludes2: symptoms, signs, and abnormal clinical laboratory findings, not elsewhere classified (R00–R99)

Rationale:

The following note appears at the beginning of Chapter 5. Therefore, it applies to all codes in the F01–F99 code range, which is the entire listing of codes in the chapter.

> *Chapter 5*
>
> *Mental and behavioral disorders (F01–F99)*
>
> *Excludes2: symptoms, signs and abnormal clinical laboratory findings, not elsewhere classified (R00–R99)*

Question 9

Correct answer:

d. Four

Rationale:

The following sequelae codes appear in the 2011 *ICD-10-CM Tabular List of Diseases and Injuries* for Chapter 6:

G09   *Sequelae of inflammatory diseases of central nervous system*

G65.0   *Sequelae of Guillain-Barré syndrome*

G65.1   *Sequelae of other inflammatory polyneuropathy*

G65.2   *Sequelae of toxic polyneuropathy*

Question 10

Correct answer:

Alzheimer's disease is classified "with early onset" and "with late onset" in Chapter 6.

Rationale:

The following are excerpts from ICD-10-CM Chapter 6:

G30.0   Alzheimer's disease with early onset

G30.1   Alzheimer's disease with late onset

Question 11

Correct answer:

b. Disorders of eye following glaucoma surgery

Rationale:

The following subcategories appear in the 2011 *ICD-10-CM Tabular List of Diseases and Injuries*:

H59.0   Disorders of the eye following cataract surgery

H59.1   Intraoperative hemorrhage and hematoma of eye and adnexa complicating a procedure

H59.2   Accidental puncture and laceration of eye and adnexa during a procedure

Question 12

Correct answer:

d. Postmastoidectomy pneumocephalus

Rationale:

No specific code exists for postmastoidectomy pneumocephalus, so code H95.88 and G93.89 should be assigned. The *ICD-10-CM Index to Diseases and Injuries* references code G93.89 for "Pneumocephalus." The *ICD-10-CM Tabular List of Diseases and Injuries* provides the code G93.89 narrative as "Other specified disorders of the brain."

There are complication codes for the other conditions:

Chronic inflammation of postmastoidectomy cavity is classified with codes H95.111–H95.119.

Granulation of postmastoidectomy cavity is classified with codes H95.121–H95.129.

Mucosal cyst of postmastoidectomy cavity is classified with codes H95.191–H95.199.

Question 13

Correct answer:

I13.0, I50.43, N18.4

Rationale:

The *ICD-10-CM Index to Diseases and Injuries* lists code I13.0.

Hypertension, hypertensive (accelerated) (benign) (essential) (idiopathic) (malignant) (systemic) I10

- cardiorenal (disease)

- - with heart failure

- - - with stage 1 through stage 4 chronic kidney disease I13.0

In the *ICD-10-CM Tabular List of Diseases and Injuries*, code I13.0 includes two "Use additional code" notes.

I13.10   Hypertensive heart and chronic kidney disease with heart failure and stage 1 through stage 4 chronic kidney disease, or unspecified chronic kidney disease

Use additional code to identify type of heart failure (I50.-)

Use additional code to identify stage of chronic kidney disease (N18.1–N18.4, N18.9)

Code I50.43 classifies the acute on chronic combined systolic congestive and diastolic congestive heart failure:

I50.43   Acute on chronic combined systolic (congestive) and diastolic (congestive) heart failure

Code N18.4 classifies the stage 4 chronic kidney disease:

N18.4   Chronic kidney disease, stage 4 (severe)

Question 14

Correct answer:

d. Code I22 should not be used if the subsequent MI occurs intraoperatively during cardiac surgery; use only code I97.790.

Rationale:

The *ICD-10-CM Index to Diseases and Injuries* references code I97.790 for an intraoperative MI.

Infarct, infarction

- myocardium, myocardial (acute) (with stated duration of four weeks or less)

- - intraoperative

- - - during cardiac surgery I97.790

Source: p. 688 of the 2011 online version of the ICD-10 manual.

In the following *ICD-10-CM Tabular List of Diseases and Injuries* excerpt, note Excludes1 prohibits the reporting of code I22 with code I97.790. When a subsequent MI occurs intraoperatively during cardiac surgery, there is a "Use additional code" note that justifies the additional reporting of code I22.

Use additional code, if applicable, to further specify disorder

I97.790 Other intraoperative cardiac functional disturbances during cardiac surgery

Question 15

Correct answer:

c. Seven

Rationale:

The following seven codes appear in Chapter 9 of the *ICD-10-CM Tabular List of Diseases and Injuries:*

I46.2	Cardiac arrest due to underlying cardiac condition
I46.8	Cardiac arrest due to other underlying condition
I46.9	Cardiac arrest, cause unspecified
I97.120	Postprocedural cardiac arrest following cardiac surgery
I97.121	Postprocedural cardiac arrest following other surgery
I97.710	Intraoperative cardiac arrest during cardiac surgery
I97.711	Intraoperative cardiac arrest during other surgery

Question 16

Correct answer:

c. Asthma

Rationale:

The *ICD-10-CM Tabular List of Diseases and Injuries*, Chapter 10, Diseases of the Respiratory System, contains the following codes for asthma:

J45.20–J45.22	Mild intermittent asthma
J45.30–J45.32	Mild persistent asthma
J45.40–J45.42	Moderate persistent asthma
J45.50–J45.52	Severe persistent asthma

Question 17

Correct answer:

K22.70   Barrett's esophagus without dysplasia

K22.710   Barrett's esophagus with low-grade dysplasia

K22.711   Barrett's esophagus with high-grade dysplasia

K22.719   Barrett's esophagus with dysplasia, unspecified

Rationale:

These codes are listed in the *ICD-10-CM Tabular List of Diseases and Injuries* under the subcategory K22.7, Barrett's esophagus. The *ICD-10-CM Index to Diseases and Injuries* also includes the term Barrett's, with esophagus and conditions indented, which includes complete diagnosis codes.

Question 18

Correct answer and rationale:

The *ICD-10-CM Index to Diseases and Injuries* lists the following:

Colitis (acute) (catarrhal) (chronic) (noninfective) (hemorrhagic) (*see also* Enteritis)

- ulcerative (chronic) <u>K51.90</u>

- - with

- - - complication <u>K51.919</u>

- - - - abscess <u>K51.914</u>

- - - - fistula <u>K51.913</u>

- - - - obstruction <u>K51.912</u>

- - - - rectal bleeding <u>K51.911</u>

- - - - specified complication necrotizing enterocolitis <u>K51.918</u>

Access the *ICD-10-CM Index to Diseases and Injuries* at *www.cms.gov/ICD10/11b1_2011_ICD10CM_and_ GEMs.asp#TopOfPage.*

Download the 2011 Code Tables and Index file.

Select icd10cm_index.

Question 19

Correct answer:

L89.321   Pressure ulcer of left buttock, stage 1

Healing pressure ulcer of left buttock, stage 1

<u>Pressure pre-ulcer skin changes limited to persistent focal edema, left buttock</u>

L89.322   Pressure ulcer of left buttock, stage 2

Healing pressure ulcer of left buttock, stage 2

<u>Pressure ulcer with abrasion, blister, partial thickness skin loss involving epidermis and/or dermis, left buttock</u>

L89.323   Pressure ulcer of left buttock, stage 3

Healing pressure ulcer of left buttock, stage 3

<u>Pressure ulcer with full thickness skin loss involving damage or necrosis of subcutaneous tissue, left buttock</u>

L89.324   Pressure ulcer of left buttock, stage 4

Healing pressure ulcer of left buttock, stage 4

<u>Pressure ulcer with necrosis of soft tissues through to underlying muscle, tendon, or bone, left buttock</u>

Rationale:

These descriptions appear in the *ICD-10-CM Tabular List of Diseases and Injuries*, Chapter 12, Diseases of the Skin and Subcutaneous Tissue.

Question 20

Correct answer:

The appropriate seventh character is to be added to each code from subcategory M84.4:

<u>A</u> - <u>initial encounter for fracture</u>

<u>D</u> - <u>subsequent encounter for fracture with routine healing</u>

G - subsequent encounter for fracture with delayed healing

K - subsequent encounter for fracture with nonunion

P - subsequent encounter for fracture with malunion

S - sequela

Rationale:

The seventh character note appears in the *ICD-10-CM Tabular List of Diseases and Injuries*, Chapter 13, Diseases of the Musculoskeletal System and Connective Tissue, below M84.4, Pathological fracture, not elsewhere classified.

Question 21

Correct answer:

Code N35.013 <u>applies to male patients only</u>

Code N35.112 <u>applies to male patients only</u>

Code N35.12 <u>applies to female patients only</u>

Code N39.3 <u>applies to both male and female patients</u>

Rationale:

The following are complete descriptions for the preceding ICD-10-CM codes:

N35.013	Post-traumatic anterior urethral stricture—this code is listed under the subcategory
N35.0	Post-traumatic urethral stricture, male
N35.112	Postinfective bulbous urethral stricture, not elsewhere classified—this code is listed under the subcategory
N35.11	Postinfective urethral stricture, not elsewhere classified, male
N35.12	Postinfective urethral stricture, not elsewhere classified, female—the code's description specifically states female
N39.3	Stress incontinence (female) (male)—the code's description specifically lists both female and male

Question 22

Correct answer:

The following code numbers and descriptions appear in the *ICD-10-CM Tabular List of Diseases and Injuries*, Chapter 15, Pregnancy, Childbirth and the Puerperium:

O03.38	Urinary tract infection following incomplete spontaneous abortion
O03.88	Urinary tract infection following complete or unspecified spontaneous abortion
O04.88	Urinary tract infection following (induced) termination of pregnancy
O07.38	Urinary tract infection following failed attempted termination of pregnancy
O08.83	Urinary tract infection following an ectopic and molar pregnancy
O86.20	Urinary tract infection following delivery, unspecified
O86.29	Other urinary tract infection following delivery

Question 23

Correct answer:

The *ICD-10-CM Index to Diseases and Injuries* lists the following:

Findings, abnormal, inconclusive, without diagnosis (see also Abnormal)

- antenatal screening of mother O28.9

- - biochemical O28.1

- - chromosomal O28.5

- - cytological O28.2

- - genetic O28.5

- - hematological O28.0

- - radiological O28.4

- - specified O28.8

- - ultrasonic O28.3

Question 24

Correct answer:

> f. Missed abortion—early fetal death before completion of 20 weeks of gestation without retention of dead fetus

Rationale:

Code O02.1, Missed abortion, in Chapter 15, Pregnancy, Childbirth and the Puerperium, in the *ICD-10-CM Tabular List of Diseases and Injuries* states:

> *Early fetal death, before completion of 20 weeks of gestation,* with retention of dead fetus.

Code O09.5, Supervision of elderly primigravida and multigravida, in Chapter 15, Pregnancy, Childbirth and the Puerperium, in the *ICD-10-CM Tabular List of Diseases and Injuries* states:

> *Pregnancy for a female 35 years and older at expected date of delivery.*

Code O09.6, Supervision of young primigravida and multigravida, in Chapter 15, Pregnancy, Childbirth and the Puerperium, in the *ICD-10-CM Tabular List of Diseases and Injuries* states:

> *Supervision of pregnancy for a female less than 16 years old at expected date of delivery.*

The note at the beginning of Chapter 15, Pregnancy, Childbirth and the Puerperium, in the *ICD-10-CM Tabular List of Diseases and Injuries* states:

> *Trimesters are counted from the first day of the last menstrual period. They are defined as follows:*
>
> > *1st trimester - less than 14 weeks 0 days*
> >
> > *2nd trimester - 14 weeks 0 days to less than 28 weeks 0 days*
> >
> > *3rd trimester - 28 weeks 0 days until delivery.*

Question 25

Correct answer:

> a. P09

Rationale:

The *ICD-10-CM Tabular List of Diseases and Injuries*, Chapter 16, Certain Conditions Originating in the Perinatal Period, indicates that code P09 is a valid code with the following description:

P09   Abnormal findings on neonatal screening

The *ICD-10-CM Tabular List of Diseases and Injuries*, Chapter 16, Certain Conditions Originating in the Perinatal Period, indicates that P10, P11, and P12 are category codes that are not valid without additional digits:

P10   Intracranial laceration and hemorrhage due to birth injury

P11   Other birth injuries to central nervous system

P12   Birth injury to scalp

Question 26

Correct answer:

False

Rationale:

The *ICD-10-CM Tabular List of Diseases and Injuries*, Chapter 16, Congenital Malformations, Deformations and Chromosomal Abnormalities, indicates that the following Excludes note applies to code Q35.5, which prohibits the reporting of codes from category Q35 with codes from category Q37:

Q35 *Cleft palate*

Excludes1: cleft palate with cleft lip (Q37.-)

Q35.1 *Cleft hard palate*

Q35.2 *Cleft soft palate*

Q35.5 *Cleft hard palate with cleft soft palate*

Q35.7 *Cleft uvula*

Q35.9 *Cleft palate, unspecified*

Question 27

Correct answer:

a. A code from subcategory R40.3 is required to complete the coma scale.

Rationale:

The *ICD-10-CM Tabular List of Diseases and Injuries*, Chapter 18, Symptoms, Signs and Abnormal Clinical and Laboratory Findings, indicates that R40.3 is a valid code and that it is not a subcategory.

R40.3   Persistent vegetative state

The *ICD-10-CM Tabular List of Diseases and Injuries*, Chapter 18, Symptoms, Signs and Abnormal Clinical and Laboratory Findings, indicates that R40.21-, R40.22-, and R40.23- are subcategories that require additional digits to be valid codes:

A note below the R40.2 Coma category states that "a code from each subcategory is required to complete the coma scale."

R40.21-   Coma scale, eyes open

R40.22-   Coma scale, best verbal response

R40.23-   Coma scale, best motor response

Question 28

Correct answer:

d. Chapter 18, Symptoms, Signs and Abnormal Clinical and Laboratory Findings

Rationale:

The *ICD-10-CM Tabular List of Diseases and Injuries*, Chapter 18, Symptoms, Signs and Abnormal Clinical and Laboratory findings, includes the following code:

R53.0   Neoplastic (malignant) related fatigue

Note: The code is listed in the index under Fatigue, neoplasm related.

Question 29

Correct answer:

<u>sequela</u>	-	avascular necrosis following fracture
<u>subsequent encounter</u>	-	cast change or removal
<u>initial encounter</u>	-	emergency treatment
<u>initial encounter</u>	-	evaluation and treatment by a new physician
<u>subsequent encounter</u>	-	follow-up visits following fracture treatment
<u>sequela</u>	-	infection on open fracture site
<u>subsequent encounter</u>	-	malunion of fracture
<u>subsequent encounter</u>	-	nonunion of fracture
<u>subsequent encounter</u>	-	medication adjustment
<u>initial encounter</u>	-	patient delayed seeking treatment for the fracture or nonunion
<u>subsequent encounter</u>	-	removal of external or internal fixation device
<u>initial encounter</u>	-	surgical treatment

Rationale:

The *ICD-10-CM Official Guidelines for Coding and Reporting 2011*, pp. 63–64, state:

> *Traumatic fractures are coded using the appropriate 7th character extension for initial encounter (A, B, C) while the patient is receiving active treatment for the fracture. Examples of active treatment are: surgical treatment, emergency department encounter, and evaluation and treatment by a new physician. The appropriate 7th character for initial encounter should also be assigned for a patient who delayed seeking treatment for the fracture or nonunion. Fractures are coded using the appropriate 7th character extension for subsequent care for encounters after the patient has completed active treatment of the fracture and is receiving routine care for the fracture during the healing or recovery phase. Examples of fracture aftercare are: cast change or removal, removal of external or internal fixation device, medication adjustment, and follow-up visits following fracture treatment. ...*
>
> *Care of complications of fractures, such as malunion and nonunion, should be reported with the appropriate 7th character extensions for subsequent care with nonunion (K, M, N) or subsequent care with malunion (P, Q, R).*

Question 30

Correct answer:

Driver: <u>An occupant of a transport vehicle who is operating or intending to operate it.</u>

Passenger: <u>Any occupant of a transport vehicle other than the driver, except a person traveling on the outside of the vehicle.</u>

Nontraffic accident: <u>Any vehicle accident that occurs entirely in any place other than a public highway.</u>

Transport accident: <u>Any accident involving a device designed primarily for, or used at the time primarily for, conveying persons or goods from one place to another.</u>

Rationale:

The *ICD-10-CM Tabular List of Diseases and Injuries* provides the preceding definitions at the beginning of Chapter 20, External Causes of Morbidity.

Question 31

Correct answer:

External cause code: Y36.230D, War operations involving explosion of improvised explosive device [IED], military personnel, subsequent encounter

External cause status code: Y99.1, Military activity

Rationale:

The *ICD-10-CM Index to Diseases and Injuries* provides the following main term and subterms to determine the final external cause status code assignment:

Status of external cause

- military activity Y99.1

In the *ICD-10-CM Index to Diseases and Injuries,* the following main term and subterms are used to obtain the tentative external cause code assignment:

"War operations (injuries to military personnel and civilians during war, civil insurrection and peacekeeping missions) (by) (from) (involving)

- explosion (of)

- - improvised explosive device [IED] (person-borne) (roadside) (vehicle-borne) Y36.23-"

The *ICD-10-CM Tabular List of Diseases and Injuries*, Chapter 20, External Causes of Morbidity, includes the following note at category Y36:

> *The appropriate 7th character is to be added to each code from category Y36*
>
> *A - initial encounter*
>
> *D - subsequent encounter*
>
> *S - sequela*

This patient is being admitted for rehabilitation therapy, which is aftercare, so the subsequent encounter seventh character extension "D" is applicable.

No place of occurrence code is assigned for subsequent encounters. This patient's initial encounter occurred at the transferring hospital. The *ICD-10-CM Tabular List of Diseases and Injuries* note for code Y92, Place of occurrence of the external cause, states:

> *Place of occurrence should be recorded only at the initial encounter for treatment.*

There is no activity code assigned on a subsequent encounter. The *ICD-10-CM Official Guidelines for Coding and Reporting 2011*, p. 73, state:

> *An activity code is used only once, at the initial encounter for treatment.*

Question 32

Correct answer:

X12.xxxA, <u>Contact with other hot fluids, initial encounter</u>

Y92.511, <u>Restaurant or café as the place of occurrence of the external cause</u>

Y93.G3, <u>Activity, cooking and baking</u>

Y99.0, <u>Civilian activity done for income or pay</u>

Rationale:

The *ICD-10-CM Index to Diseases and Injuries* includes the following main term and subterms to determine the tentative external cause code assignment:

Burn, burned, burning (accidental) (by) (from) (on)

- hot

- - liquid NEC X12

The *ICD-10-CM Tabular List of Diseases and Injuries*, Chapter 20, External Causes of Morbidity, includes the following note at code X12:

> *The appropriate 7th character is to be added to code X12*
>
> *A - initial encounter*
>
> *D - subsequent encounter*
>
> *S - sequela*

This patient is being seen in the emergency department, so the initial encounter seventh character extension "A" is applicable.

In the *ICD-10-CM Index to Diseases and Injuries*, the following main term and subterms are used to obtain the place of occurrence, activity, and external cause status code assignments:

Place of occurrence

- restaurant Y92.511

Activity (involving) (of victim at time of event)

- cooking and baking Y93.G3

Status of external cause

- civilian activity done for income or pay Y99.0

Question 33

Correct answer:

The following code numbers and descriptions appear in the *ICD-10-CM Tabular List of Diseases and Injuries*, Chapter 21, Factors Influencing Health status and Contact with Health Services:

Z00.01   Encounter for general adult medical examination with abnormal findings

Z00.121   Encounter for routine child health examination with abnormal findings

<u>Z00.71</u>   <u>Encounter for examination for period of delayed growth in childhood with abnormal findings</u>

<u>Z01.01</u>   <u>Encounter for examination of eyes and vision with abnormal findings</u>

<u>Z01.21</u>   <u>Encounter for dental examination and cleaning with abnormal findings</u>

<u>Z01.31</u>   <u>Encounter for examination of blood pressure with abnormal findings</u>

<u>Z01.411</u>   <u>Encounter for gynecological examination (general) (routine) with abnormal findings</u>

Question 34

Correct answer:

b. Drug dependence

Rationale:

ICD-10-CM does not include a code that denotes a personal history of drug dependence. The *ICD-10-CM Index to Diseases and Injuries* classifies personal history of drug dependence to drug dependence in remission, which is not a personal history code.

History

- personal (of)

- - drug dependence—*see* Dependence, drug, by type, in remission

The *ICD-10-CM Tabular List of Diseases and Injuries*, Chapter 21, Factors Influencing Health Status and Contact with Health Services, indicates that the other conditions have specific personal history codes:

Z87.710   Personal history of (corrected) hypospadias

Z87.81   Personal history of (healed) traumatic fracture

Z86.31   Personal history of diabetic foot ulcer

Question 35

Correct answer:

The following code numbers and descriptions appear in the *ICD-10-CM Tabular List of Diseases and Injuries,* Chapter 21, Factors Influencing Health Status and Contact with Health Services:

Z08   Encounter for follow-up examination after completed treatment for malignant neoplasm

Z09   Encounter for follow-up examination after completed treatment for conditions other than malignant neoplasm

Z16   Infection with drug-resistant microorganisms

Z21   Asymptomatic human immunodeficiency virus [HIV] infection status

Z23   Encounter for immunization

Z36   Encounter for antenatal screening of mother

Z66   Do not resuscitate

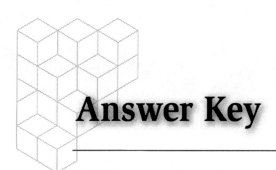
Answer Key

Case Study 1

Correct answer:

S51.012A   Laceration without foreign body of left elbow

S51.012A   Laceration without foreign body of left elbow

S81.812A   Laceration without foreign body, left lower leg

I48.0   Atrial fibrillation

M06.9   Rheumatoid arthritis, unspecified

R32   Unspecified urinary incontinence

K21.9   Gastroesophageal reflux disease without esophagitis

W10.0XXA   Fall (on) (from) escalator

Y92.520   Airport as the place of occurrence of the external cause

Y99.8   Other external cause status

Rationale:

For the left elbow lacerations, the *ICD-10-CM Index to Diseases and Injuries* provides the tentative code S51.01-:

Laceration

- elbow S51.01-

A review of code S51.01 in the *ICD-10-CM Tabular List of Diseases and Injuries* provides the incomplete code S51.012:

> S51.012   Laceration without foreign body of left elbow

The following note in the *ICD-10-CM Tabular List of Diseases and Injuries* indicates that code S51.012 is incomplete because a seventh character is required:

> *Add the appropriate 7th character to each code from category S51:*
>
> *A - initial encounter*
>
> *D - subsequent encounter*
>
> *S - sequela*

Based on documentation in the visit note, the final code is:

> S51.012A   Laceration without foreign body of left elbow

The *ICD-10-CM Official Guidelines for Coding and Reporting*, p. 62, state:

> *Extension "A," initial encounter is used while the patient is receiving active treatment for the injury. Examples of active treatment are: surgical treatment, emergency department encounter, and evaluation and treatment by a new physician.*

The *ICD-10-CM Index to Diseases and Injuries* provides the tentative code S81.812 for the left shin laceration:

> Laceration
>
> - shin—*see* Laceration, leg

> Laceration
>
> - leg (lower)
>
> - - left S81.812

A review of code S81.812 in the *ICD-10-CM Tabular List of Diseases and Injuries* provides the incomplete code S81.812:

> S81.812   Laceration without foreign body, left lower leg

The following note in the *ICD-10-CM Tabular List of Diseases and Injuries* indicates that code S81.812 is incomplete because a seventh character is required:

The appropriate 7th character is to be added to each code from category S81:

A - initial encounter

D - subsequent encounter

S - sequela

Based on documentation in the visit note, the final code is:

S81.812A   Laceration without foreign body, left lower leg

The *ICD-10-CM Official Guidelines for Coding and Reporting 2011*, p. 62, state:

Extension "A", initial encounter is used while the patient is receiving active treatment for the injury. Examples of active treatment are: surgical treatment, emergency department encounter, and evaluation and treatment by a new physician.

Refer to the *ICD-10-CM External Cause of Injuries Index* for the fall down the escalator stairs:

Fall, falling (accidental)

- in, on

- - escalator W10.0

A review of code W10.0 in the *ICD-10-CM Tabular List of Diseases and Injuries* provides the incomplete code W10.0:

W10.0   Fall (on) (from) escalator

The following note in the *ICD-10-CM Tabular List of Diseases and Injuries* indicates that code W10.0 is incomplete because a seventh character is required:

The appropriate 7th character is to be added to each code from category W10:

A - initial encounter

D - subsequent encounter

S - sequela

Based on documentation in the visit note, the final code is:

W10.0XXA   Fall (on) (from) escalator

The *ICD-10-CM Official Guidelines for Coding and Reporting 2011*, p. 62, state:

Extension "A", initial encounter is used while the patient is receiving active treatment for the injury. Examples of active treatment are: surgical treatment, emergency department encounter, and evaluation and treatment by a new physician.

Refer to *ICD-10-CM External Cause of Injuries Index* for the airport location of the fall:

Place of occurrence

- airport Y92.520

A review of code Y92.520 in the *ICD-10-CM Tabular List of Diseases and Injuries* confirms that this is an accurate and complete code:

Y92.520   Airport as the place of occurrence of the external cause

Refer to the *ICD-10-CM External Cause of Injuries Index* to code the patient's status (i.e., visitor from Texas):

Status of external cause

- leisure activity Y99.8

A review of code Y99.8 in the *ICD-10-CM Tabular List of Diseases and Injuries* confirms that this is an accurate and complete code:

Y99.8   Other external cause status

The patient was traveling (she had arrived at her airport destination) when she fell. Because there is no specific ICD-10-CM activity code for traveling, no Y93 code is assigned for this case. The *ICD-10-CM Official Guidelines for Coding and Reporting 2011*, p. 73, state:

A code from category Y93 is appropriate for use with external cause and intent codes if identifying the activity provides additional information about the event.

The following *ICD-10-CM Index to Diseases and Injuries* entries support the other conditions listed as "illnesses" for which the patient is taking medications:

The *ICD-10-CM Official Guidelines for Coding and Reporting 2011*, p. 98, state:

> Code all documented conditions that coexist at the time of the encounter/visit, and require or affect patient care treatment or management. Do not code conditions that were previously treated and no longer exist. However, history codes (categories Z80–Z87) may be used as secondary codes if the historical condition or family history has an impact on current care or influences treatment.

Hypothyroidism (acquired) E03.9

Fibrillation

- atrial or auricular (established) I48.0

Arthritis, arthritic (acute) (chronic) (nonpyogenic) (subacute)

- rheumatoid M06.9

M06.9   Rheumatoid arthritis, unspecified

Coding Note: Rheumatoid arthritis has expanded to site and laterality for ICD-10-CM.

Incontinence R32

R32   Unspecified urinary incontinence

Coding Note: Check the Excludes1 note for R32.

Reflux

gastroesophageal K21.9

Case Study 2

Correct Answer:

N39.0	Urinary tract infection, site not specified
N99.89	Other postprocedural complications and disorders of genitourinary system
R31.9	Hematuria, unspecified
M54.5 5	Lumbago, NOS
Y83.8	Other surgical procedures as the cause of abnormal reaction of the patient, or of later complication, without mention of misadventure at the time of the procedure

Rationale:

For the urinary tract infection, the *ICD-10-CM Index to Diseases and Injuries* provides the following code:

Infection, infected, infective (opportunistic)

- urinary (tract) N39.0

The *ICD-10-CM Index to Diseases and Injuries* provides the tentative code for hematuria secondary to laser transurethral procedure:

Complication(s) (from) (of)

- postprocedural—*see also* Complications, surgical procedure

- - specified NEC

- - - genitourinary N99.89

Because the hematuria is not classified in code N99.89, use the *ICD-10-CM Index to Diseases and Injuries* to locate the tentative code for hematuria:

Hematuria R31.9

Coding Note: Excludes2 provides hematuria NOS (R31-), recurrent or persistent hematuria (N02.-)

Refer to the *ICD-10-CM External Cause of Injuries Index* for laser transurethral procedure as the external cause of hematuria:

Complication (delayed) of or following (medical or surgical procedure)

- surgical operation

- - specified NEC Y83.8

The *ICD-10-CM Index to Diseases and Injuries* provides the following code for low back pain, musculoskeletal:

Pain(s) (*see also* Painful)

- musculoskeletal (*see also* Pain, by site) M79.1

- back (postural) M54.9

- low back (M54.5)

A review of code M54.5 in the *ICD-10-CM Tabular List of Diseases and Injuries* confirms that this is an accurate and complete code:

M54.5 Low back pain

　　　Lumbago

Coding Note: Refer to the Excludes1 note regarding strain, due to intervertebral disc displacement, and "lumbago with sciatica."

Coding Application Note: Cross review of code M79.1 = Myofascial pain syndrome.

Case Study 3

Correct answer:

I21.09	ST elevation myocardial infarction (STEMI) involving other coronary artery of anterior wall
I25.10	Atherosclerotic heart disease of native coronary artery without angina pectoris
E11.9	Type 2 diabetes mellitus without complications
E78.5	Hyperlipidemia, unspecified
Z95.1	Presence of aortocoronary bypass graft
Z79.4	Long-term (current) use of insulin

Rationale:

For the anterior wall myocardial infarction, the *ICD-10-CM Index to Diseases and Injuries* provides the following code:

Infarct, infarction

- - ST elevation (STEMI)

- - - anterior (anteroapical) (anterolateral) (anteroseptal) (Q wave) (wall) I21.09

The following *ICD-10-CM Index to Diseases and Injuries* entries support the other conditions listed as "illnesses" for which the patient is taking medications and/or impact treatment of the patient:

Disease, diseased—*see also* Syndrome

- artery

- - coronary I25.10

Diabetes, diabetic (mellitus) (sugar) E11.9

E11.9   Type 2 diabetes mellitus without complications

Z79.4   Long-term (current) use of insulin

Coding Note: In the tabular section, under the E11 Type 2 diabetes mellitus subcategory, refer to the "Use additional code to identify any insulin use (Z79.4)."

Hyperlipemia, hyperlipidemia E78.5

Status (post)—*see also* Presence (of)

- aortocoronary bypass Z95.1

The *ICD-10-CM Official Guidelines for Coding and Reporting 2011*, p. 98, state:

Code all documented conditions that coexist at the time of the encounter/visit, and require or affect patient care treatment or management. Do not code conditions that were previously treated and no longer exist. However, history codes (categories Z80–Z87) may be used as secondary codes if the historical condition or family history has an impact on current care or influences treatment.

Case Study 4

Correct answer:

      S20.221A   Contusion of right back wall of thorax

      I10   Essential (primary) hypertension

      E78.5   Hyperlipidemia, unspecified

Rationale:

For the back/chest wall contusion, the *ICD-10-CM Index to Diseases and Injuries* provides the tentative code:

      Contusion (skin surface intact)

      - back—*see also* Contusion, thorax, back

      - chest (wall)—*see* Contusion, thorax

      - thorax (wall)

      - - back S20.22-

Coding Application Note: Notice in the S20.2- category for contusion of thorax, front wall and back wall, with laterality was added for ICD-10-CM.

A review of code S20.22- in the *ICD-10-CM Tabular List of Diseases and Injuries* provides this incomplete code:

      S20.221   Contusion of right back wall of thorax

The following note in the *ICD-10-CM Tabular List of Diseases and Injuries* indicates that code S20.221 is incomplete because a seventh character is required:

      The appropriate 7th character is to be added to each code from category S20

      A - initial encounter

      D - subsequent encounter

      S - sequela

Based on documentation in the visit note, the final code is:

      S20.221A   Contusion of right back wall of thorax

The *ICD-10-CM Official Guidelines for Coding and Reporting 2011*, p. 62, state:

Extension "A", initial encounter is used while the patient is receiving active treatment for the injury. Examples of active treatment are: surgical treatment, emergency department encounter, and evaluation and treatment by a new physician.

The following *ICD-10-CM Index to Diseases and Injuries* entries support the other conditions listed as "illnesses" for which the patient is taking medications:

Hyperlipemia, hyperlipidemia E78.5

Hypertension, hypertensive (accelerated) (benign) (essential) (idiopathic) (malignant) (systemic) I10

The *ICD-10-CM Official Guidelines for Coding and Reporting 2011*, p. 98, state:

Code all documented conditions that coexist at the time of the encounter/visit, and require or affect patient care treatment or management. Do not code conditions that were previously treated and no longer exist. However, history codes (categories Z80-Z87) may be used as secondary codes if the historical condition or family history has an impact on current care or influences treatment.

Case Study 5

Correct answer:

F41.8   Anxiety depression (mild or not persistent)

F43.10   Post-traumatic stress disorder, unspecified

Z91.410   Personal history of adult physical and sexual abuse

Rationale:

The *ICD-10-CM Index to Diseases and Injuries* provides the following code for anxiety depression:

Depression (acute) (mental) F32.9

- Anxiety F41.8

Anxiety F41.9

- depression F41.8

Coding Application Note: "Persistent" (F34.1) was not documented

F41.8   Other specified anxiety disorders

Anxiety depression, anxiety hysteria, and mixed anxiety and depressive disorder

The *ICD-10-CM Index to Diseases and Injuries* provides the following code for PTSD:

Disorder (of)—*see also* Disease

- post-traumatic stress (PTSD) F43.10

Coding Application Note: The F43.10–F43.12 codes are categorized in the tabular section also by unspecified (F43.10), acute (F43.11), and chronic (F43.12).

The following *ICD-10-CM Index to Diseases and Injuries* entry supports the patient's history of physical abuse by her ex-husband:

History

- personal (of)

- - abuse

- - - adult

- - - - physical and sexual Z91.410

The *ICD-10-CM Official Guidelines for Coding and Reporting 2011*, p. 98, state:

Code all documented conditions that coexist at the time of the encounter/visit, and require or affect patient care treatment or management. Do not code conditions that were previously treated and no longer exist. However, history codes (categories Z80–Z87) may be used as secondary codes if the historical condition or family history has an impact on current care or influences treatment.

Case Study 6

Correct answer:

F31.9   Bipolar disorder, unspecified

F41.1   Generalized anxiety disorder

F60.89   Other specific personality disorders

I10   Essential (primary) hypertension

E11.9   Type 2 diabetes mellitus without complications

Z63.8   Other specified problems related to primary support group

Z59.9   Problem related to housing and economic circumstances, unspecified

Rationale:

The *ICD-10-CM Index to Diseases and Injuries* provides the following code for bipolar I disorder, most recent episode depressed:

Disorder (of)

- bipolar (I) F31.9

- - current episode

- - - depressed F31.9

The *ICD-10-CM Index to Diseases and Injuries* provides the following code for the generalized anxiety disorder:

Disorder (of)

- anxiety

- - generalized F41.1

The *ICD-10-CM Index to Diseases and Injuries* provides no specific reference for the cluster B personality disorder, so use the following code:

Disorder (of)

- personality (*see also* Personality)

- - specified NEC F60.89

The *ICD-10-CM Index to Diseases and Injuries* provides the following code for hypertension:

Hypertension, hypertensive (accelerated) (benign) (essential) (idiopathic) (malignant) (systemic) I10

The *ICD-10-CM Index to Diseases and Injuries* provides the following code for diabetes mellitus type 2:

Diabetes, diabetic (mellitus) (sugar)

- type 2 E11.9

The *ICD-10-CM Index to Diseases and Injuries* provides the following code for family discord:

Discord (with)

- family Z63.8

Because code Z63.8 includes "Inadequate family support NOS," it also includes the patient's lack of social support.

The *ICD-10-CM Index to Diseases and Injuries* provides the following code for financial issues:

Problem (with) (related to)

- finance Z59.9

Case Study 7

Correct answer:

Z00.00	Encounter for general adult medical examination without abnormal findings
F20.0	Paranoid schizophrenia
Z72.0	Tobacco use
N39.3	Stress incontinence (female) (male)
E66.9	Obesity, unspecified
Z68.32	Body mass index (BMI) 32.0–32.9, adult

Rationale:

The reason for the visit is the healthcare maintenance/general physical exam. The *ICD-10-CM Index to Diseases and Injuries* provides the following code:

Examination (for) (following) (general) (of) (routine)

- medical (adult) (for) (of) Z00.00

The *ICD-10-CM Index to Diseases and Injuries* provides the following code for paranoid schizophrenia:

Schizophrenia, schizophrenic

- paranoid (type) F20.0

The *ICD-10-CM Index to Diseases and Injuries* provides the following code for tobacco abuse:

Use (of)

- tobacco Z72.0

The *ICD-10-CM Index to Diseases and Injuries* provides the following code for stress incontinence:

Incontinence

- stress (female) (male) N39.3

In the review of systems, the physician states that the patient is obese and documents her body mass index.

The *ICD-10-CM Index to Diseases and Injuries* provides the following code for obesity:

Obesity E66.9

The *ICD-10-CM Index to Diseases and Injuries* provides the following code for a body mass index of 32.5:

Body, bodies

- mass index (BMI)

- - adult

- - - 32.0–32.9 Z68.32

The *ICD-10-CM Official Guidelines for Coding and Reporting 2011*, p. 98, state:

Code all documented conditions that coexist at the time of the encounter/visit, and require or affect patient care treatment or management. Do not code conditions that were previously treated and no longer exist. However, history codes (categories Z80–Z87) may be used as secondary codes if the historical condition or family history has an impact on current care or influences treatment.

Case Study 8

Correct answer:

Z00.00	Encounter for general adult medical examination without abnormal findings
N31.9	Neuromuscular dysfunction of bladder, unspecified
G80.9	Cerebral palsy, unspecified

Rationale:

The *ICD-10-CM Index to Diseases and Injuries* provides the following code for the healthcare maintenance/general physical exam:

Examination (for) (following) (general) (of) (routine)

- medical (adult) (for) (of) Z00.00

The *ICD-10-CM Index to Diseases and Injuries* provides the following code for the neurogenic bladder:

Neurogenic—*see also* condition

- bladder (*see also* Dysfunction, bladder, neuromuscular) N31.9

The *ICD-10-CM Index to Diseases and Injuries* provides the following code for cerebral palsy:

Palsy (*see also* Paralysis)

- cerebral (congenital) G80.9

Case Study 9

Correct answer:

J18.9	Pneumonia, unspecified organism
R79.89	Other specified abnormal findings of blood chemistry
D64.9	Anemia, unspecified
E78.0	Pure hypercholesterolemia
N40.0	Enlarged prostate without lower urinary tract symptoms (LUTS)
Z95.1	Presence of aortocoronary bypass graft

Z96.652   Presence of left artificial knee joint

Z86.73   Personal history of transient ischemic attack (TIA), and cerebral infarction without residual deficits

I25.2   Old myocardial infarction

Rationale:

The *ICD-10-CM Index to Diseases and Injuries* provides the following code for left lower lobe pneumonia:

Pneumonia (acute) (Alpenstich) (benign) (bilateral) (brain) (cerebral) (circumscribed) (congestive) (creeping) (delayed resolution) (double) (epidemic) (fever) (flash) (fulminant) (fungoid) (granulomatous) (hemorrhagic) (incipient) (infantile) (infectious) (infiltration) (insular) (intermittent) (latent) (migratory) (organized) (overwhelming) (primary (atypical) progressive) (pseudolobar) (purulent) (resolved) (secondary) (senile) (septic) (suppurative) (terminal) (true) (unresolved) (vesicular) J18.9

The *ICD-10-CM Index to Diseases and Injuries* provides the following code for elevated myoglobin:

Abnormal, abnormality, abnormalities

- chemistry, blood

- - specified NEC R79.89

The *ICD-10-CM Index to Diseases and Injuries* provides the following code for anemia:

Anemia (essential) (general) (hemoglobin deficiency) (infantile) (primary) (profound) D64.9

The following *ICD-10-CM Index to Diseases and Injuries* entries support the other conditions listed under past medical history that affect the patient's treatment or for which the patient is currently taking medications:

Elevated, elevation

- cholesterol E78.0

Enlargement, enlarged—*see also* Hypertrophy

- prostate N40.0

Status (post)—*see also* Presence (of)

- aortocoronary bypass Z95.1

Presence (of)

- knee-joint implant (functional) (prosthesis) Z96.65-

History

- personal (of)

- - transient ischemic attack (TIA) without residual deficits Z86.73

History

- personal (of)

- - myocardial infarction (old) I25.2

The *ICD-10-CM Official Guidelines for Coding and Reporting 2011*, p. 98, state:

> *Code all documented conditions that coexist at the time of the encounter/visit, and require or affect patient care treatment or management. Do not code conditions that were previously treated and no longer exist. However, history codes (categories Z80–Z87) may be used as secondary codes if the historical condition or family history has an impact on current care or influences treatment.*

Case Study 10

Correct answer:

G89.21	Chronic pain due to past trauma
M54.2	Cervicalgia
G43.909	Migraine, unspecified, not intractable, without status migrainosus
G89.4	Chronic pain syndrome
W10.9xxS	Fall (on) (from) unspecified stairs and steps

Rationale:

The *ICD-10-CM Index to Diseases and Injuries* provides the following code for chronic cervical neck pain (which began after a fall down a flight of stairs three years ago):

Pain(s)

- chronic

- - due to trauma G89.21

The ICD-10-CM *Tabular List of Diseases and Injuries* at category G89 includes an Excludes2 note that requires coding of the neck pain:

Excludes2: localized pain, unspecified type - code to pain by site, such as: spine pain (M54.-)

The *ICD-10-CM Index to Diseases and Injuries* provides the following code:

Pain(s)

- neck NEC M54.2

The *ICD-10-CM Index to Diseases and Injuries* provides the following code for migraine headaches:

Headache

- migraine (type) (*see also* Migraine) G43.909

The *ICD-10-CM Index to Diseases and Injuries* provides the following code for chronic pain syndrome:

Syndrome

- chronic

- - pain G89.4

The *ICD-10-CM External Cause of Injuries Index* provides the tentative code for the fall down a flight of stairs three years ago:

Fall, falling (accidental)

- down

- - stairs, steps W10.9

The *ICD-10-CM Tabular List of Diseases and Injuries* provides the incomplete code W10.9:

W10.9   Fall (on) (from) unspecified stairs and steps

The following note in the *ICD-10-CM Tabular List of Diseases and Injuries* indicates that code W10.9 is incomplete because a seventh character is required:

Add the appropriate 7th character to each code from category W10

A - initial encounter

D - subsequent encounter

S - sequela

Based on documentation in the visit note, the final code is:

W10.9xxS   Fall (on) (from) unspecified stairs and steps

The *ICD-10-CM Official Guidelines for Coding and Reporting 2011*, p. 75, state:

Late effects are reported using the external cause code with the 7th character extension "S" for sequela. These codes should be used with any report of a late effect or sequela resulting from a previous injury.

Case Study 11

Correct answer:

B94.8   Sequelae of other specified infectious and parasitic diseases

R22.2   Localized swelling, mass and lump, trunk

R11.2   Nausea with vomiting, unspecified

F31.9   Bipolar disorder, unspecified

G43.909   Migraine, unspecified, not intractable, without status migrainosus

Note: There is no documentation that the hydrocephalus is still being treated or that the ventriculoperitoneal shunt is still in place.

Rationale:

The *ICD-10-CM Index to Diseases and Injuries* provides the following code for resolving herpes zoster (with red bumps that are burning):

Sequelae (of)—*see also* condition

- infectious disease B94.9

- - specified NEC B94.8

The following notes appear in the *ICD-10-CM Tabular List of Diseases and Injuries* in section "Sequelae of infectious and parasitic diseases (B90-B94)":

Note: Categories B90-B94 are to be used to indicate conditions in categories A00-B89 as the cause of sequelae, which are themselves classified elsewhere. The 'sequelae' include conditions specified as such; they also include residuals of diseases classifiable to the above categories if there is evidence that the disease itself is no longer present. Codes from these categories are not to be used for chronic infections. Code chronic current infections to active infectious disease as appropriate.

Code first condition resulting from (sequela) the infectious or parasitic disease.

Because the burning red bumps on her chest are a condition resulting from herpes zoster, the *ICD-10-CM Index to Diseases and Injuries* is referenced and provides the following code:

Mass

- localized (skin) R22.9

- - trunk R22.2

For nausea with vomiting (viral gastroenteritis rather than Zyprexa® side effects), the *ICD-10-CM Index to Diseases and Injuries* provides the following code:

Nausea (without vomiting)

- with vomiting R11.2

The *ICD-10-CM Official Guidelines for Coding and Reporting 2011*, p. 98, state:

Do not code diagnoses documented as "probable," "suspected," "questionable," "rule out," or "working diagnosis" or other similar terms indicating uncertainty. Rather, code the condition(s) to the highest degree of certainty for that encounter/visit, such as symptoms, signs, abnormal test results, or other reason for the visit.

The following *ICD-10-CM Index to Diseases and Injuries* entries support the other conditions listed under medical history for which the patient is currently receiving medication:

Disorder (of)

- bipolar (I) F31.9

Migraine (idiopathic) G43.909

The *ICD-10-CM Official Guidelines for Coding and Reporting 2011*, p. 98, state:

Code all documented conditions that coexist at the time of the encounter/visit, and require or affect patient care treatment or management. Do not code conditions that were previously treated and no longer exist. However, history codes (categories Z80–Z87) may be used as secondary codes if the historical condition or family history has an impact on current care or influences treatment.

Case Study 12

Correct answer:

G43.909   Migraine, unspecified, not intractable, without status migrainosus

Z91.128   Patient's intentional underdosing of medication regimen for other reason

S69.92xD   Unspecified injury of left wrist, hand and finger(s)

Z86.71   Personal history of venous thrombosis and embolism

W19.xxxD   Unspecified fall

Rationale:

The *ICD-10-CM Index to Diseases and Injuries* provides the following code for a migraine headache:

Headache

- migraine (type) (*see also* Migraine) G43.909

The *ICD-10-CM Index to Diseases and Injuries* provides the following code to denote that the patient does not have the medications that she usually has (secondary to insurance issues):

Underdosing

- intentional NEC Z91.128

The *ICD-10-CM Index to Diseases and Injuries* provides the following incomplete code for a left wrist injury:

Injury

- wrist S69.9-

A review of the *ICD-10-CM Tabular List of Diseases and Injuries* provides this incomplete code:

S69.92   Unspecified injury of left wrist, hand, and finger(s)

The following note in the *ICD-10-CM Tabular List of Diseases and Injuries* indicates that code S69.92 is incomplete because a seventh character is required:

The appropriate 7th character is to be added to each code from category S69:

A - initial encounter

D - subsequent encounter

S - sequela

Based on documentation in the visit note (i.e., splint is on her left wrist secondary to a fall she sustained about a week ago, and she was given prescription for a second set of x-rays), the final code is:

S69.92xD   Unspecified injury of left wrist, hand, and finger(s)

The *ICD-10-CM Official Guidelines for Coding and Reporting 2011*, p. 62, state:

*Extension "D" subsequent encounter is used for encounters after the patient has received active treatment of the injury and is receiving routine care for the injury during the healing or recovery phase. Examples of subsequent care are: cast change or removal, removal of external **or** internal fixation device, medication adjustment, other aftercare and follow up visits following injury treatment.*

For the fall onto her outstretched hand which she sustained about a week ago, see the *ICD-10-CM External Cause of Injuries Index*:

Fall, falling (accidental) W19

A review of code W19 in the *ICD-10-CM Tabular List of Diseases and Injuries* provides the incomplete code W19:

W19   Unspecified fall

The following note in the *ICD-10-CM Tabular List of Diseases and Injuries* indicates that code W19 is incomplete because a seventh character is required:

The appropriate 7th character is to be added to each code from category W19:

A - initial encounter

D - subsequent encounter

S - sequela

Based on documentation in the visit note, the final code is:

W19.xxxD   Unspecified fall

The *ICD-10-CM Official Guidelines for Coding and Reporting 2011*, p. 62, state:

> *Assign the external cause code, with the appropriate 7th character (initial encounter, subsequent encounter or sequela) for each encounter for which the injury or condition is being treated.*

The *ICD-10-CM Index to Diseases and Injuries* provides the following code for a history of pulmonary embolism:

History

- personal (of)

- - embolism (venous) Z86.71

Case Study 13

Correct answer:

I10	Essential (primary) hypertension
I69.193	Ataxia following nontraumatic intracerebral hemorrhage
I69.198	Other sequelae of nontraumatic intracerebral hemorrhage
R20.0	Anesthesia of skin
E78.5	Hyperlipidemia, unspecified
R45.4	Irritability and anger

Rationale:

For the hypertension, the *ICD-10-CM Index to Diseases and Injuries* provides the following code:

> Hypertension, hypertensive (accelerated) (benign) (essential) (idiopathic) (malignant) (systemic) I10

The *ICD-10-CM Index to Diseases and Injuries* provides the following code for the recent hemorrhagic cerebrovascular accident with gradual resolution of his symptoms (some trouble with fine motor movements of the right hand):

Sequelae (of)

- hemorrhage

- - intracerebral

- - - ataxia I69.193

The *ICD-10-CM Index to Diseases and Injuries* provides the following code for the recent hemorrhagic cerebrovascular accident with gradual resolution of his symptoms (some numbness in his thumb):

Sequelae (of)

- hemorrhage

- - intracerebral

- - - alteration of sensation I69.198

The *ICD-10-CM Tabular List of Diseases and Injuries*, at code I69.198 indicates that there is a "Use additional code" note:

Use additional code to identify the sequelae.

Because numbness in the thumb requires an additional code, the *ICD-10-CM Index to Diseases and Injuries* is referenced for the following code:

Numbness R20.0

The *ICD-10-CM Index to Diseases and Injuries* provides the following code for hyperlipidemia:

Hyperlipemia, hyperlipidemia E78.5

The *ICD-10-CM Index to Diseases and Injuries* provides the following code difficulty with stress and anger management:

Anger R45.4

Case Study 14

Correct answer:

S93.402   Sprain of unspecified ligament of left ankle

M81.0   Age-related osteoporosis without current pathological fracture

E78.5   Hyperlipidemia, unspecified

I10   Essential (primary) hypertension

E03.9   Hypothyroidism, unspecified

W18.49xA   Other slipping, tripping, and stumbling without falling

Rationale:

The *ICD-10-CM Index to Diseases and Injuries* provides the following incomplete code a left ankle sprain:

Sprain (joint) (ligament)

- ankle S93.40-

Based on documentation in the visit note and a review of code S93.40- in the *ICD-10-CM Tabular List of Diseases and Injuries*, the final code is:

S93.402   Sprain of unspecified ligament of left ankle

Refer to the *ICD-10-CM External Cause of Injuries Index* for the slipping and twisted ankle:

Slipping (accidental) (on same level) (with fall) W01.0

- without fall W18.40

- - due to

- - - specified NEC W18.49

A review of code W18.49 in the *ICD-10-CM Tabular List of Diseases and Injuries* provides the incomplete code:

W18.49   Other slipping, tripping, and stumbling without falling

The following note in the *ICD-10-CM Tabular List of Diseases and Injuries* indicates that code W18.49 is incomplete because a seventh character is required:

The appropriate 7th character is to be added to each code from category W18:

A - initial encounter

D - subsequent encounter

S - sequela

Based on documentation in the visit note, the final code is:

W18.49xA   Other slipping, tripping, and stumbling without falling

The *ICD-10-CM Official Guidelines for Coding and Reporting 2011*, p. 62, state:

"Extension "A", initial encounter is used while the patient is receiving active treatment for the injury. Examples of active treatment are: surgical treatment, emergency department encounter, and evaluation and treatment by a new physician.

Because the location of her injury (e.g., house, apartment, hotel room) is not documented, there is no place of occurrence code to assign.

Refer to the *ICD-10-CM External Cause of Injuries Index* to code the patient's status (i.e., visiting from Birmingham):

Status of external cause

- leisure activity Y99.8

A review of code Y99.8 in the *ICD-10-CM Tabular List of Diseases and Injuries* confirms that this is an accurate and complete code:

Y99.8   Other external cause status

- Activity NEC

- - Leisure activity

The patient was running to answer the telephone when she fell, which is not the same as running for exercise or relaxation. Because there is no specific ICD-10-CM activity code for attempting to answer a telephone while traveling, no Y93 code is assigned for this case.

The *ICD-10-CM Official Guidelines for Coding and Reporting 2011*, p. 73, state:

> *A code from category Y93 is appropriate for use with external cause and intent codes if identifying the activity provides additional information about the event.*

The following *ICD-10-CM Index to Diseases and Injuries* entries support the other conditions listed under past medical history for which the patient is taking medications and/or impact treatment of the patient:

Osteoporosis (female) (male) M81.0

Hyperlipemia, hyperlipidemia E78.5

Hypertension, hypertensive (accelerated) (benign) (essential) (idiopathic) (malignant) (systemic) I10

Hypothyroidism (acquired) E03.9

The *ICD-10-CM Official Guidelines for Coding and Reporting 2011*, p. 98, state:

> *Code all documented conditions that coexist at the time of the encounter/visit, and require or affect patient care treatment or management. Do not code conditions that were previously treated and no longer exist. However, history codes (categories Z80–Z87) may be used as secondary codes if the historical condition or family history has an impact on current care or influences treatment.*

Case Study 15

Correct answer:

M06.9	Rheumatoid arthritis, unspecified
M85.80	Other specified disorders of bone density and structure, unspecified site
J62.8	Pneumoconiosis due to other dust containing silica
R63.6	Underweight
Z68.1	Body mass index (BMI) 19 or less, adult
Z87.891	Personal history of nicotine dependence

Rationale:

For the rheumatoid arthritis, the *ICD-10-CM Index to Diseases and Injuries* provides the following code:

Arthritis, arthritic (acute) (chronic) (nonpyogenic) (subacute)

- rheumatoid M06.9

The *ICD-10-CM Index to Diseases and Injuries* provides the following code for osteopenia:

Osteopenia M85.8-

For the chronic obstructive pulmonary disease secondary to Kaplan's syndrome/pulmonary silicosis, the *ICD-10-CM Index to Diseases and Injuries* provides the following codes:

Silicosis, silicotic (simple) (complicated) J62.8

and

Disease, diseased

- lung

- - obstructive (chronic) J44.9

Code J44.9 (Chronic obstructive pulmonary disease, unspecified) cannot be assigned with code J62.8 for this case because an Excludes1 note at category J44 states:

Excludes1: lung diseases due to external agents (J60-J70)

The *ICD-10-CM Index to Diseases and Injuries* provides the following code for underweight:

Underweight R63.6

Because underweight is a diagnosis and body mass index (BMI) 16.5 is provided, the *ICD-10-CM Index to Diseases and Injuries* is referenced for the following code:

Body, bodies

- mass index (BMI)

- - adult

- - - 19 or less Z68.1

Because the patient was "previously a smoker," the *ICD-10-CM Index to Diseases and Injuries* is referenced for the following code:

History

- personal (of)

- - tobacco dependence Z87.891

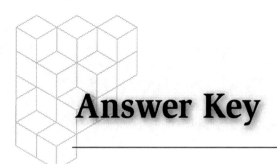

Chapter 3

Answer Key

Question 1

Correct answer:

c. The biopsy is coded along with a repair (root operation) code for the site at which the definitive procedure was performed.

Rationale:

In *ICD-10-PCS Coding Guidelines 2011*, guideline B3.4 states:

If a diagnostic Excision, Extraction, or Drainage procedure (biopsy) is followed by a more definitive procedure, such as Destruction, Excision or Resection at the same procedure site, both the biopsy and the more definitive treatment are coded.

Question 2

Correct answer:

High: <u>Amputation at the proximal portion of the shaft of the humerus or femur</u>

Mid: <u>Amputation at the middle portion of the shaft of the humerus or femur</u>

Low: <u>Amputation at the distal portion of the shaft of the humerus or femur</u>

Rationale:

ICD-10-PCS Reference Manual 2011 lists the previous definitions on p. 2.13.

Access the *ICD-10-PCS Reference Manual 2011* at *www.cms.gov/ICD10/11b_2011_ICD10PCS. asp#TopOfPage.*

Select 2011 ICD-10 Reference Manual and Slides.

Select I10_Coding_ref_11.

Question 3

Correct answer:

Bone marrow and endometrial biopsies are not coded to the root operation excision; they are coded to the root operation <u>extraction</u> with the qualifier <u>diagnostic</u>.

Rationale:

ICD-10-PCS Reference Manual 2011, p. 2.9, states:

> *Bone marrow and endometrial biopsies are not coded to Excision, they are coded to Extraction, with the Qualifier Diagnostic.*

Question 4

Correct answer:

The root operation <u>repair</u> also functions as the "not elsewhere classified (NEC)" root operation to be used when the medical and surgical procedure performed does not meet the definition of one of the other root operations.

Rationale:

ICD-10-PCS Reference Manual 2011, p. 2.64, states:

> *The root operation REPAIR represents a broad range of procedures for restoring the anatomic structure of a body part such as suture of lacerations. REPAIR also functions as the "not elsewhere classified (NEC)" root operation, to be used when the procedure performed does not meet the definition of one of the other root operations.*

Question 5

Correct answer:

Severing a nerve root to relieve pain is coded to the root operation division.

Rationale:

Guideline B3.14 in the *ICD-10-PCS Coding Guidelines 2011* states:

> *If the sole objective of the procedure is freeing a body part without cutting the body part, the root operation is Release. If the sole objective of the procedure is separating or transecting a body part, the root operation is Division.*

> *Examples: Freeing a nerve root from surrounding scar tissue to relieve pain is coded to the root operation Release. Severing a nerve root to relieve pain is coded to the root operation Division.*

Question 6

Correct answer:

c. Removal

Rationale:

ICD-10-PCS Reference Manual 2011, p. A.7, states:

> *A Removal procedure is coded for taking out the device used in a previous replacement procedure.*

Question 7

Correct answer:

d. Resection, excision

Rationale:

ICD-10-PCS Reference Manual 2011, p. 2.11, states:

> *When an entire lymph node chain is cut out, the appropriate root operation is RESECTION.*
> *When a lymph node(s) is cut out, the root operation is EXCISION.*

Question 8

Correct answer:

b. Coded to the root operation performed

Rationale:

ICD-10-PCS Reference Manual 2011, p. 2.58, states:

A complete re-do of a medical and surgical procedure is coded to the root operation performed.

Question 9

Correct answer:

a. The body system value; The qualifier

Rationale:

ICD-10-PCS Reference Manual 2011, p. 2.35, states:

The body system value describes the deepest tissue layer in the flap. The qualifier can be used to describe the other tissue layers, if any, being transferred.

Question 10

Correct answer:

c. Kidney

Rationale:

Guideline B4.1b in the *ICD-10-PCS Coding Guidelines 2011* states:

If the prefix "peri" is combined with a body part to identify the site of the procedure, the procedure is coded to the body part named.

Example: A procedure site identified as perirenal is coded to the kidney body part.

Question 11

Correct answer:

> c. The most distal body part inspected is coded

Rationale:

> Guideline B3.11b in the *ICD-10-PCS Coding Guidelines 2011* states:
>
> > *If multiple tubular body parts are inspected, the most distal body part inspected is coded. If multiple non-tubular body parts in a region are inspected, the body part that specifies the entire area inspected is coded.*

Question 12

Correct answer:

> c. Administration

Rationale:

> *ICD-10-PCS Reference Manual 2011*, p. 2.32, states:
>
> > *Bone marrow transplant procedures are coded in section 3 Administration to the root operation 2 Transfusion.*

Question 13

Correct answer:

> c. Individuals or tissues that have identical genes, such as identical twins

Rationale:

> The following definitions explain how these processes differ:
>
> > Allogeneic: Tissues taken from different individuals of the same species
> >
> > Syngeneic: Individuals or tissues that have identical genes, such as identical twins
> >
> > Zooplastic: Tissues transferred from an animal to a human

Question 14

Correct answer:

5A1221Z and 5A1935Z

Rationale:

Cardiopulmonary bypass takes over two functions of the body, so two codes are necessary: the first for taking over the function of the heart and the second for the lungs.

FIGURE 3.1

Cardiopulmonary Bypass

Performance defines procedures where complete control is exercised over a physiological function, such as total mechanical ventilation, cardiac pacing, and cardiopulmonary bypass.

Example: Cardiopulmonary bypass in conjunction with CABG

Character 1 Section	Character 2 Body System	Character 3 Root Operation	Character 4 Body System	Character 5 Duration	Character 6 Function	Character 7 Qualifier
EXTRACORP. ASSISTANCE & PERFORMANCE	PHYSIOLOGICAL SYSTEMS	PERFORMANCE	CARDIAC	CONTINUOUS	OUTPUT	NO QUALIFIER
5	A	1	2	2	1	Z

Character 1 Section	Character 2 Body System	Character 3 Root Operation	Character 4 Body System	Character 5 Duration	Character 6 Function	Character 7 Qualifier
EXTRACORP. ASSISTANCE & PERFORMANCE	PHYSIOLOGICAL SYSTEMS	PERFORMANCE	RESPIRATORY	LESS THAN 24 CONSEC. HRS	VENTILATION	NO QUALIFIER
5	A	1	9	3	5	Z

Source: Adapted from ICD-10-PCS Reference Manual 2011, *p. 3.15.*

Access the ICD-10-PCS Reference Manual 2011 *at www.cms.gov/ICD10/11b_2011_ICD10PCS.asp#TopOfPage.*

Select 2011 ICD-10-PCS Reference Manual and Slides.

Select I10_Coding_ref_11.

This technique uses a heart-lung machine to continuously maintain perfusion to other body organs and tissues during surgery (i.e., mechanically circulates and oxygenates blood from the body while bypassing the heart and lungs).

ICD-10-PCS Reference Manual 2011, p. 3.15.

Question 15

Correct answer:

False

Rationale:

ICD-10-PCS Reference Manual 2011, p. 3.15, states:

> *Restoration defines only external cardioversion and defibrillation procedures. Failed cardio-version procedures are also included in the definition of Restoration, and are coded the same as successful procedures.*

Question 16

Correct answer:

False

Rationale:

Guideline B3.01b in the *ICD-10-PCS Coding Guidelines 2011* states:

> *If multiple vertebral joints are fused, a separate procedure is coded for each vertebral joint that uses a different device and/or qualifier.*

Question 17

Correct answer:

> a. The definition of abortion is artificially terminating a pregnancy before 20 completed weeks of gestation

Rationale:

The ICD-10-PCS definition of the root operation abortion does not include the duration of a pregnancy The *ICD-10-PCS Reference Manual 2011*, p. 3.5, states:

> *Abortion. Artificially terminating a pregnancy.*

> *Delivery. Assisting the passage of the products of conception from the genital canal.*

> *Abortion is subdivided according to whether an additional device such as a laminaria or abortifacient is used, or whether the abortion was performed by mechanical means.*

> *If either a laminaria or abortifacient is used, then the approach is Via Natural or Artificial Opening.*

> *All other abortion procedures are those done by mechanical means (the products of conception are physically removed using instrumentation), and the device value is Z, no device.*

Question 18

Correct answer:

> b. No bilateral body part value exists for the nasal turbinates, so each procedure is coded separately using the appropriate nasal turbinate body part value

Rationale:

Guideline B4.3 in the *ICD-10-PCS Coding Guidelines 2011* states:

> *Bilateral body part values are available for a limited number of body parts. If the identical procedure is performed on contralateral body parts, and a bilateral body part value exists for that body part, a single procedure is coded using the bilateral body part value. If no bilateral body part value exists, each procedure is coded separately using the appropriate body part value.*

Question 19

Correct answer:

Anterior intercostals artery

Internal thoracic artery

Musculophrenic artery

Pericardiophrenic artery

Superior epigastric artery

Rationale:

"Definitions, Medical and Surgical – Body Part," *ICD-10-CM PCS Code Tables and Index 2011* PDF file, p. 1092.

FIGURE 3.2

Section 0 - Medical and Surgical Character 4 - Body Part

	Includes:
Internal Mammary Artery, Left Internal Mammary Artery, Right	Anterior intercostal artery Internal thoracic artery Musculophrenic artery Pericardiophrenic artery Superior epigastric artery

Source: Adapted from ICD-10 Procedure Coding System (ICD-10-PCS) 2011 Tables and Index.

Access the ICD-10 Procedure Coding System (ICD-10-PCS) 2011 Tables and Index at www.cms.gov/ICD10/11b_2011_ICD10PCS.asp#TopOfPage.

Select 2011 Code Tables and Index.

Question 20

Correct answer:

c. Cervical vertebral joint

Rationale:

"Definitions, Medical and Surgical – Body Part," *ICD-10-CM PCS Code Tables and Index 2011* PDF file, p. 1082.

FIGURE 3.3

Section 0 - Medical and Surgical Character 4 - Body Part

Cervical Vertebral Joint	**Includes:** Atlantoaxial joint Cervical facet joint

Source: Adapted from ICD-10 Procedure Coding System (ICD-10-PCS) 2011 Tables and Index.

Access the ICD-10 Procedure Coding System (ICD-10-PCS) 2011 Tables and Index at www.cms.gov/ICD10/11b_2011_ICD10PCS.asp#TopOfPage.

Select 2011 Code Tables and Index.

Question 21

Correct answer:

Coronary arteries are classified by number of <u>distinct sites treated</u>, rather than number of coronary arteries or anatomic name of a coronary artery (e.g., left anterior descending).

The <u>body part</u> identifies the number of coronary artery sites bypassed <u>to</u>.

The <u>qualifier</u> specifies the vessel bypassed <u>from</u>.

Rationale:

Guideline B3.6b in the *ICD-10-PCS Coding Guidelines 2011* states:

> *Coronary arteries are classified by number of distinct sites treated, rather than number of coronary arteries or anatomic name of a coronary artery (e.g., left anterior descending). Coronary artery bypass procedures are coded differently than other bypass procedures as described in the previous guideline. Rather than identifying the body part bypassed from, the body part identifies the number of coronary artery sites bypassed to, and the qualifier specifies the vessel bypassed from.*

Question 22

Correct answer:

c. In the other procedures section, there is a specific method for "robotic-assisted procedure"

Rationale:

In the ICD-10-PCS Index, the following main term and subterms direct users to the other procedures root operation table 8E0, which lists method value "C Robotics Assisted Procedure."

Robotic Assisted Procedure

Extremity

Lower 8E0Y

Upper 8E0X

Head and Neck Region 8E09

Trunk Region 8E0W

8EO

Section	8 Other Procedures
Body System	E Physiological Systems and Anatomical Regions
Operation	0 Other Procedures: Methodologies which attempt to remediate or cure a disorder or disease

Body Region	Approach	Method	Qualifier
1 Nervous System U Female Reproductive System	X External	Y Other Method	7 Examination
2 Circulatory System	3 Percutaneous	D Near Infrared Spectroscopy	Z No Qualifier
9 Head and Neck Region W Trunk Region	0 Open 3 Percutaneous 4 Percutaneous Endoscopic 7 Via Natural or Artificial Opening 8 Via Natural or Artificial Opening Endoscopic	C Robotic Assisted Procedure	Z No Qualifier
9 Head and Neck Region W Trunk Region	X External	B Computer Assisted Procedure	F With Fluoroscopy G With Computerized Tomography H With Magnetic Resonance Imaging Z No Qualifier
9 Head and Neck Region W Trunk Region	X External	C Robotic Assisted Procedure	Z No Qualifier
9 Head and Neck Region W Trunk Region	X External	Y Other Method	8 Suture Removal
H Integumentary System and Breast	3 Percutaneous	0 Acupuncture	0 Anesthesia Z No Qualifier
H Integumentary System and Breast	X External	6 Collection	2 Breast Milk
H Integumentary System and Breast	X External	Y Other Method	9 Piercing
K Musculoskeletal System	X External	1 Therapeutic Massage	Z No Qualifier
K Musculoskeletal System	X External	Y Other Method	7 Examination
V Male Reproductive System	X External	1 Therapeutic Massage	C Prostate D Rectum
V Male Reproductive System	X External	6 Collection	3 Sperm

FIGURE 3.4

8EO (cont.)

Body Region	Approach	Method	Qualifier
X Upper Extremity **Y** Lower Extremity	**0** Open **3** Percutaneous **4** Percutaneous Endoscopic	**C** Robotic Assisted Procedure	**Z** No Qualifier
X Upper Extremity **Y** Lower Extremity	**X** External	**C** Computer Assisted Procedure	**F** With Fluoroscopy **G** With Computerized Tomography **H** Magnetic Resonance Imaging **Z** No Qualifier
X Upper Extremity **Y** Lower Extremity	**X** External	**C** Robotic Assisted Procedure	**Z** No Qualifier
X Upper Extremity **Y** Lower Extremity	**X** External	**Y** Other Method	**8** Suture Removal

Source: Adapted from ICD-10 Procedure Coding System (ICD-10-PCS) 2011 Tables and Index.

Access the ICD-10 Procedure Coding System (ICD-10-PCS) 2011 Tables and Index at www.cms.gov/ICD10/11b_2011_ICD10PCS.asp#TopOfPage.

Select 2011 Code Tables and Index.

Question 23

Correct answer:

Casting of a nondisplaced fracture is coded to the root operation <u>immobilization</u> in the <u>placement</u> section. Putting in a pin in a nondisplaced fracture is coded to the root operation <u>insertion</u>. Closed reduction of a displaced fracture is coded to the root operation <u>reposition</u>.

Rationale:

Guideline B3.15 in the *ICD-10-PCS Coding Guidelines 2011* states:

> *Reduction of a displaced fracture is coded to the root operation Reposition and the application of a cast or splint in conjunction with the Reposition procedure is not coded separately. Treatment of a nondisplaced fracture is coded to the procedure performed.*

Examples: Putting a pin in a nondisplaced fracture is coded to the root operation Insertion.

Casting of a nondisplaced fracture is coded to the root operation Immobilization in the Placement section.

Question 24

Correct answer:

Cardiac catheterization:	<u>Measurement</u>
Cesarean section:	<u>Extraction</u>
Latissimus dorsi myocutaneous flap:	<u>Replacement</u>
Mechanical ventilation:	<u>Performance</u>
Quarantine:	<u>Other procedures</u>

Rationale:

In the ICD-10-PCS Index, the following main term and subterms direct users to the appropriate root operation table, which includes the name and definition of the root operation:

Caesarean section *see* Extraction, Products of Conception 10D0

Mechanical ventilation *see* Performance, Respiratory 5A19

Quarantine 8E0ZXY6

Latissimus Dorsi Myocutaneous Flap

   Bilateral 0HRV075

   Left 0HRU075

   Right 0HRT075

Catheterization

   Heart *see* Measurement, Cardiac 4A02

Question 25

Correct answer and rationale:

The ICD-10-PCS Index lists the following main term and subterms.

Transfusion

    Vein

        Central

            Antihemophilic factors <u>3024</u>

               Blood

                  Platelets <u>3024</u>

                  Red cells <u>3024</u>

                    Frozen <u>3024</u>

                  White cells <u>3024</u>

                  Whole <u>3024</u>

               Bone marrow <u>3024</u>

Question 26

Correct answer:

a. If the intended procedure is discontinued use the "discontinued procedure" qualifier as the seventh character.

Rationale:

ICD-10-PCS does not include a discontinued procedure qualifier.

Guideline B3.3 in the *ICD-10-PCS Coding Guidelines 2011* states:

If the intended procedure is discontinued, code the procedure to the root operation performed.
If a procedure is discontinued before any other root operation is performed, code the root operation Inspection of the body part or anatomical region inspected.

Question 27

Correct answer:

c. Via natural or artificial opening endoscopic

Rationale:

"Definitions, Medical and Surgical–Approach," *ICD-10-CM PCS Code Tables and Index 2011*
PDF file, p. 1115:

> *Via Natural or Artificial Opening Endoscopic. Definition: Entry of instrumentation through a natural or artificial external opening to reach and visualize the site of the procedure.*

> *Pouchoscopy is a procedure that allows your physician to examine the lining of your ileo-anal pouch for inflammation, abnormal growths or tissue. An ileo-anal pouch is a surgically created pouch to replace the colon and rectum. During a pouchoscopy, the doctor inserts a flexible tube called an endoscope into the anus and advances it slowly into the pouch. If abnormal tissue is found, the doctor may remove a sample for further examination or biopsy.*
> Source: *www.mngastro.com/tests-amp-procedures/tests-and-procedures/pouchoscopy*

Question 28

Correct answer:

False

Rationale:

In root table 02H, seventh value "S" is not in the same row as the first six characters, so this is not a valid code.

ICD-10-PCS Reference Manual 2011, p. 1.13, states:

> *A table may be separated into rows to specify the valid choices of values in characters 4 through 7. A code built using values from more than one row of a table is not a valid code.*

| FIGURE 3.5 | | | 02H |

Section	**0** Medical and Surgical
Body System	**2** Heart and Great Vessels
Operation	**H** Insertion: Putting in a nonbiological appliance that monitors, assists, performs, or prevents a physiological function but does not physically take the place of a body part.

Body Part	Approach	Device	Qualifier
4 Coronary Vein **6** Atrium, Right **7** Atrium, Left **K** Ventricle, Right **L** Ventricle, Left	**0** Open **3** Percutaneous **4** Percutaneous Endoscopic	**2** Monitoring Device	**G** Pressure Sensor **Z** No Qualifier
4 Coronary Vein **6** Atrium, Right **7** Atrium, Left **K** Ventricle, Right **L** Ventricle, Left	**0** Open **3** Percutaneous **4** Percutaneous Endoscopic	**3** Infusion Device **D** Intraluminal Device	**Z** No Qualifier
4 Coronary Vein **6** Atrium, Right **7** Atrium, Left **K** Ventricle, Right **L** Ventricle, Left	**0** Open **3** Percutaneous **4** Percutaneous Endoscopic	**M** Cardiac Lead	**A** Pacemaker Lead **E** Defibrillator Lead **Z** No Qualifier
A Heart	**0** Open **3** Percutaneous **4** Percutaneous Endoscopic	**Q** Implantable Heart Assist System	**Z** No Qualifier
A Heart	**0** Open **3** Percutaneous **4** Percutaneous Endoscopic	**R** External Heart Assist System	**S** Biventricular **Z** No Qualifier
N Pericardium	**0** Open **3** Percutaneous **4** Percutaneous Endoscopic	**2** Monitoring Device	**G** Pressure Sensor **Z** No Qualifier
N Pericardium	**0** Open **3** Percutaneous **4** Percutaneous Endoscopic	**M** Cardiac Lead	**A** Pacemaker Lead **E** Defibrillator Lead **Z** No Qualifier

FIGURE 3.5			02H (cont.)

Body Part	Approach	Device	Qualifier
P Pulmonary Trunk **Q** Pulmonary Artery, Right **R** Pulmonary Artery, Left **S** Pulmonary Vein, Right **T** Pulmonary Vein, Left **V** Superior Vena Cava **W** Thoracic Aorta	**0** Open **3** Percutaneous **4** Percutaneous Endoscopic	**2** Monitoring Device	**G** Pressure Sensor **Z** No Qualifier
P Pulmonary Trunk **Q** Pulmonary Artery, Right **R** Pulmonary Artery, Left **S** Pulmonary Vein, Right **T** Pulmonary Vein, Left **V** Superior Vena Cava **W** Thoracic Aorta	**0** Open **3** Percutaneous **4** Percutaneous Endoscopic	**3** Infusion Device **D** Intraluminal Device	**Z** No Qualifier

Source: Adapted from ICD-10 Procedure Coding System (ICD-10-PCS) 2011 Tables and Index.

Access the ICD-10 Procedure Coding System (ICD-10-PCS) 2011 Tables and Index at www.cms.gov/ICD10/11b_2011_ICD10PCS.asp#TopOfPage.

Select 2011 Code Tables and Index.

Question 29

Correct answer:

b. Value, characters

Rationale:

ICD-10-PCS Reference Manual 2011, p. 1.6, states:

> *All codes in ICD-10-PCS are seven characters long. Each character in the seven-character code represents an aspect of the procedure. . . . The process consists of assigning values from among the valid choices for that part of the system, according to the rules governing the construction of codes. . . . This code is derived by choosing a specific value for each of the seven characters.*

Question 30

Correct answer:

Shoulder <u>is coded to upper arm</u>

Elbow <u>is coded to lower arm</u>

Wrist <u>is coded to lower arm</u>

Hip <u>is coded to upper leg</u>

Knee <u>is coded to lower leg</u>

Ankle <u>is coded to foot</u>

Rationale:

Guideline B4.6 in the *ICD-10-PCS Coding Guidelines 2011* states:

> *If a procedure is performed on the skin, subcutaneous tissue or fascia overlying a joint, the procedure is coded to the following body part:*
>
> *Shoulder is coded to Upper Arm*
>
> *Elbow is coded to Lower Arm*
>
> *Wrist is coded to Lower Arm*
>
> *Hip is coded to Upper Leg*
>
> *Knee is coded to Lower Leg*
>
> *Ankle is coded to Foot.*

Question 31

Correct answer:

h. Placement

Rationale:

Placement is not listed as a root operation in the "Definitions, Obstetrics - Operation," *ICD-10-CM PCS Code Tables and Index 2011* PDF file, pp. 1116–1118.

Question 32

Correct answer:

False

Rationale:

Guideline B6.1a in the *ICD-10-PCS Coding Guidelines 2011* states:

A device is coded only if a device remains after the procedure is completed. If no device remains, the device value No Device is coded. (The guideline does not specify the type of device.)

Question 33

Correct answer:

c. Resection of a joint is performed during joint replacement surgery

Rationale:

Guideline B3.1b in the *ICD-10-PCS Coding Guidelines 2011* states:

Resection of a joint as part of a joint replacement procedure is included in the root operation definition of Replacement and is not coded separately. (Guideline B3.2 allows reporting of the other scenarios listed.)

Question 34

Correct answer:

PCS contains specific body parts for anatomical subdivisions of a body part, such as lobes of the lungs or liver and regions of the intestine. Resection of the specific body part is coded whenever all of the body part is cut out or off, rather than coding excision of a less specific body part.

Rationale:

Guideline B3.8 of the *ICD-10-PCS Coding Guidelines 2011*.

Question 35

Correct answer:

Procedures performed following a delivery or abortion for curettage of the endometrium or evacuation of retained products of conception are all coded in the <u>obstetrics</u> section, to the root operation <u>extraction</u>, and the body part <u>products of conception, retained</u>.

Rationale:

Guideline C2 of the *ICD-10-PCS Coding Guidelines 2011* states:

Procedures performed following a delivery or abortion for curettage of the endometrium or evacuation of retained products of conception are all coded in the Obstetrics section, to the root operation Extraction and the body part Products of Conception, Retained.

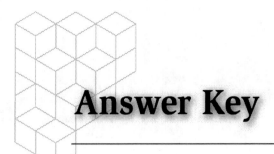

Chapter 4

Answer Key

Case Study 1

Correct answer:

> 0D160ZA
>
> 0WHF33Z
>
> 3E0M3BZ

Rationale:

> The Billroth II procedure is also called gastrojejunostomy. It involves the partial gastrectomy (or removal of the antrum and pylorus of stomach) with anastomosis of the gastric stump to the jejunum.

> For a gastrojejunostomy, the ICD-10-PCS Index references the first four characters of the 0D1 root operation table:

> > Gastrojejunostomy
> >
> > *see* Bypass, Stomach 0D16

> A review of the 0D1 root operation table and the operative report provides the information needed to assign the remaining three characters of the code:

Section:	0	Medical and surgical
Body system:	D	Gastrointestinal system
Operation:	1	Bypass: Altering the route of passage of the contents of a tubular body part

Body part: 6   Stomach

Approach: 0   Open (a laparotomy was performed as the surgical approach)

Device: Z   No device (the stomach was anastomosed directly to the jejunum
                           without an interposing graft)

Qualifier: A   Jejunum (jejunum was secured to the posterior wall of the stomach)

FIGURE 4.1

0D1

Section	0 Medical and Surgical
Body System	D Gastrointestinal System
Operation	1 Bypass: Altering the route of passage of the contents of a tubular body part

Body Part	Approach	Device	Qualifier
1 Esophagus, Upper 2 Esophagus, Middle 3 Esophagus, Lower 5 Esophagus	0 Open 4 Percutaneous Endoscopic 8 Via Natural or Artificial Opening Endoscopic	7 Autologous Tissue Substitute J Synthetic Substitute K Nonautologous Tissue Substitute Z No Device	4 Cutaneous 6 Stomach 9 Duodenum A Jejunum B Ileum
1 Esophagus, Upper 2 Esophagus, Middle 3 Esophagus, Lower 5 Esophagus	3 Percutaneous	J Synthetic Substitute	4 Cutaneous
6 Stomach 9 Duodenum	0 Open 4 Percutaneous Endoscopic 8 Via Natural or Artificial Opening Endoscopic	7 Autologous Tissue Substitute J Synthetic Substitute K Nonautologous Tissue Substitute Z No Device	4 Cutaneous 9 Duodenum A Jejunum B Ileum L Transverse Colon
6 Stomach 9 Duodenum	3 Percutaneous	J Synthetic Substitute	4 Cutaneous
A Jejunum	0 Open 4 Percutaneous Endoscopic 8 Via Natural or Artificial Opening Endoscopic	7 Autologous Tissue Substitute J Synthetic Substitute K Nonautologous Tissue Substitute Z No Device	4 Cutaneous A Jejunum B Ileum H Cecum K Ascending Colon L Transverse Colon M Descending Colon N Sigmoid Colon P Rectum Q Anus

FIGURE 4.1

0D1 (cont.)

Body Part	Approach	Device	Qualifier
A Jejunum	**3** Percutaneous	**J** Synthetic Substitute	**4** Cutaneous
B Ileum	**0** Open **4** Percutaneous Endoscopic **8** Via Natural or Artificial Opening Endoscopic	**7** Autologous Tissue Substitute **J** Synthetic Substitute **K** Nonautologous Tissue Substitute **Z** No Device	**4** Cutaneous **A** Jejunum **B** Ileum **H** Cecum **K** Ascending Colon **L** Transverse Colon **M** Descending Colon **N** Sigmoid Colon **P** Rectum **Q** Anus
B Ileum	**3** Percutaneous	**J** Synthetic Substitute	**4** Cutaneous
H Cecum	**0** Open **4** Percutaneous Endoscopic **8** Via Natural or Artificial Opening Endoscopic	**7** Autologous Tissue Substitute **J** Synthetic Substitute **K** Nonautologous Tissue Substitute **Z** No Device	**4** Cutaneous **H** Cecum **K** Ascending Colon **L** Transverse Colon **M** Descending Colon **N** Sigmoid Colon **P** Rectum
H Cecum	**3** Percutaneous	**J** Synthetic Substitute	**4** Cutaneous
K Ascending Colon	**0** Open **4** Percutaneous Endoscopic **8** Via Natural or Artificial Opening Endoscopic	**7** Autologous Tissue Substitute **J** Synthetic Substitute **K** Nonautologous Tissue Substitute **Z** No Device	**4** Cutaneous **K** Ascending Colon **M** Descending Colon **N** Sigmoid Colon **P** Rectum
K Ascending Colon	**3** Percutaneous	**J** Synthetic Substitute	**4** Cutaneous
L Transverse Colon	**0** Open **4** Percutaneous Endoscopic **8** Via Natural or Artificial Opening Endoscopic	**7** Autologous Tissue Substitute **J** Synthetic Substitute **K** Nonautologous Tissue Substitute **Z** No Device	**4** Cutaneous **L** Transverse Colon **M** Descending Colon **N** Sigmoid Colon **P** Rectum
L Transverse Colon	**3** Percutaneous	**J** Synthetic Substitute	**4** Cutaneous

FIGURE 4.1

0D1 (cont.)

Body Part	Approach	Device	Qualifier
M Descending Colon	**0** Open **4** Percutaneous Endoscopic **8** Via Natural or Artificial Opening Endoscopic	**7** Autologous Tissue Substitute **J** Synthetic Substitute **K** Nonautologous Tissue Substitute **Z** No Device	**4** Cutaneous **M** Descending Colon **N** Sigmoid Colon **P** Rectum
M Descending Colon	**3** Percutaneous	**J** Synthetic Substitute	**4** Cutaneous
N Sigmoid Colon	**0** Open **4** Percutaneous Endoscopic **8** Via Natural or Artificial Opening Endoscopic	**7** Autologous Tissue Substitute **J** Synthetic Substitute **K** Nonautologous Tissue Substitute **Z** No Device	**4** Cutaneous **N** Sigmoid Colon **P** Rectum
N Sigmoid Colon	**3** Percutaneous	**J** Synthetic Substitute	**4** Cutaneous

Source: Adapted from ICD-10 Procedure Coding System (ICD-10-PCS) 2011 Tables and Index.

Access the ICD-10 Procedure Coding System (ICD-10-PCS) 2011 Tables and Index at www.cms.gov/ICD10/11b_2011_ICD10PCS.asp#TopOfPage.

Select 2011 Code Tables and Index.

ON-Q® pain pump is a drug delivery system used for postoperative pain management.

The Coding Clinic for ICD-9-CM, published by the American Hospital Association in the second quarter of 2000, states:

> *The PainBuster system is a self-contained external elastometric drug delivery system that is being used for postoperative pain management. The new system alleviates pain by delivering anesthetics (i.e., Novocaine) directly into the surgical site. The system is compact and portable and includes an introducer needle, catheter, elastometric infusion pump, and an administration set, which controls the flow rate.*

> *During the placement of the PainBuster system, the surgeon inserts a catheter into the wound. The pump is then attached externally and infuses anesthetics at a preset flow rate. Patients can be discharged with the system intact for continuous therapeutic drug delivery.*

Note: There is currently no way in ICD-10-PCS to code the attachment of the catheter to the external pump. The extracorporeal therapy and other procedure sections of ICD-10-PCS do not apply for the connection of an external pump to a percutaneously placed catheter.

For the insertion of the ON-Q® pump catheter into the wound (on each side of the abdominal wall), the ICD-10-PCS Index references the first four characters of the 0WH root operation table:

Insertion of device in abdominal wall 0WHF

A review of the 0WH root operation table and the operative report provides the information needed to assign the remaining three characters of the code:

Section:	0	Medical and surgical
Body system:	W	Anatomical regions, general
Operation:	H	Insertion: putting in a nonbiological appliance that monitors, assists, performs, or prevents a physiological function but does not physically take the place of a body part
Body part:	F	Abdominal wall
Approach:	3	Percutaneous (the catheter was advanced through a sheath)
Device:	3	Infusion device (the catheter is part of the continuous drug delivery system)
Qualifier:	Z	No qualifier

FIGURE 4.2

0WH

Section	**0**	Medical and Surgical
Body System	**W**	Anatomical Regions, General
Operation	**H**	Insertion: Putting in a nonbiological appliance that monitors, assists, performs, or prevents a physiological function but does not physically take the place of a body part

Body Part	Approach	Device	Qualifier
0 Head **1** Cranial Cavity **2** Face **3** Oral Cavity and Throat **4** Upper Jaw **5** Lower Jaw **6** Neck **8** Chest Wall **9** Pleural Cavity, Right **B** Pleural Cavity, Left **C** Mediastinum **D** Pericardial Cavity **F** Abdominal Wall **G** Peritoneal Cavity **H** Retroperitoneum **J** Pelvic Cavity **K** Upper Back **L** Lower Back **M** Perineum, Male **N** Perineum, Female	**0** Open **3** Percutaneous **4** Percutaneous Endoscopic	**1** Radioactive Element **3** Infusion Device **Y** Other Device	**Z** No Qualifier
P Gastrointestinal Tract **Q** Respiratory Tract **R** Genitourinary Tract	**0** Open **3** Percutaneous **4** Percutaneous Endoscopic **7** Via Natural or Artificial Opening **8** Via Natural or Artificial Opening Endoscopic	**1** Radioactive Element **3** Infusion Device **Y** Other Device	**Z** No Qualifier

Source: Adapted from ICD-10 Procedure Coding System (ICD-10-PCS) 2011 Tables and Index.

Access the ICD-10 Procedure Coding System (ICD-10-PCS) 2011 Tables and Index at www.cms.gov/ICD10/11b_2011_ICD10PCS.asp#TopOfPage.

Select 2011 Code Tables and Index.

For the infusion of Marcaine® 0.5% via the ON-Q® pump, the ICD-10-PCS Index references all seven characters of the 3E0 root operation table:

Introduction

Peritoneal cavity

Anesthetic, local 3E0M3BZ

A review of the 03E root operation table and the operative report provides the information needed to verify the accuracy of the code:

Section:	3	Administration
Body system:	E	Physiological systems and anatomical regions
Operation:	0	Introduction: putting in or on a therapeutic, diagnostic, nutritional, physiological, or prophylactic substance except blood or blood products
Body system/ region:	M	Peritoneal cavity (the anesthetic is being infused into the laparotomy wound cavity; a laparotomy involves making an incision into the patient's abdomen to divide skin and connective tissue [called fascia], and the lining of the abdominal cavity [the peritoneum] is cut)
Approach:	3	Percutaneous (the anesthetic is administered via a catheter that was placed via a sheath and an external pump)
Substance:	B	Local anesthetic
Qualifier:	Z	No qualifier

FIGURE 4.3

3E0

Section	**3**	Administration
Body System	**E**	Physiological Systems and Anatomical Regions
Operation	**0**	Introduction: Putting in or on a therapeutic, diagnostic, nutritional, physiological, or prophylactic substance except blood or blood products

Body System/Region	Approach	Device	Qualifier
L Pleural Cavity **M** Peritoneal Cavity	**0** Open	**5** Adhesion Barrier	**Z** No Qualifier
L Pleural Cavity **M** Peritoneal Cavity	**3** Percutaneous	**0** Antineoplastic	**4** Liquid Brachytherapy Radioisotope **5** Other Antineoplastic **M** Monoclonal Antibody
L Pleural Cavity **M** Peritoneal Cavity	**3** Percutaneous	**2** Anti-infective	**8** Oxazolidinones **9** Other Anti-infective
L Pleural Cavity **M** Peritoneal Cavity	**3** Percutaneous	**3** Anti-inflammatory **6** Nutritional Substance **7** Electrolytic and Water Balance Substance **B** Local Anesthetic **H** Radioactive Substance **J** Contrast Agent **K** Other Diagnostic Substance **N** Analgesics, Hypnotics, Sedatives **T** Destructive Agent	**Z** No Qualifier
L Pleural Cavity **M** Peritoneal Cavity	**3** Percutaneous	**G** Other Therapeutic Substance	**C** Other Substance
L Pleural Cavity **M** Peritoneal Cavity	**3** Percutaneous	**S** Gas	**F** Other Gas
L Pleural Cavity **M** Peritoneal Cavity	**7** Via Natural or Artificial Opening	**0** Antineoplastic	**4** Liquid Brachytherapy Radioisotope **5** Other Antineoplastic **M** Monoclonal Antibody
L Pleural Cavity **M** Peritoneal Cavity	**7** Via Natural or Artificial Opening	**S** Gas	**F** Other Gas

Source: Adapted from ICD-10 Procedure Coding System (ICD-10-PCS) 2011 Tables and Index.

Access the ICD-10 Procedure Coding System (ICD-10-PCS) 2011 Tables and Index at www.cms.gov/ICD10/11b_2011_ICD10PCS.asp#TopOfPage.

Select 2011 Code Tables and Index.

Case Study 2

Correct answer:

10E0XZZ

0WQN0ZZ

Rationale:

For a normal spontaneous vaginal delivery, the ICD-10-PCS Index references all seven characters of the 10E root operation table:

Delivery

Manually assisted 10E0XZZ

A review of the 10E root operation table and the delivery report provides the information needed to verify the code:

Section:	1	Obstetrics
Body system:	0	Pregnancy
Operation:	E	Delivery: Assisting the passage of the products of conception from the genital canal
Body part:	0	Products of conception
Approach:	X	External
Device:	Z	No device
Qualifier:	Z	No qualifier

FIGURE
4.4

10E

Section	**1** Obstetrics
Body System	**0** Pregnancy
Operation	**E** Delivery: Assisting the passage of the products of conception from the genital canal

Body Part	Approach	Device	Qualifier
0 Products of Conception	**X** External	**Z** No Device	**Z** No Qualifier

Source: Adapted from ICD-10 Procedure Coding System (ICD-10-PCS) 2011 Tables and Index.

Access the ICD-10 Procedure Coding System (ICD-10-PCS) 2011 Tables and Index at www.cms.gov/ICD10/11b_2011_ ICD10PCS.asp#TopOfPage.

Select 2011 Code Tables and Index.

For the suture repair of the first degree laceration of the perineum, the ICD-10-PCS Index references the first four characters of the 0WQ root operation table:

Repair:

    Perineum Female 0WQN

A review of the 0WQ root operation table and the operative report provides the information needed to assign the remaining three characters of the code:

Section:	0	Medical and surgical
Body system:	W	Anatomical regions, general
Operation:	Q	Repair: restoring, to the extent possible, a body part to its normal anatomic structure and function
Body part:	N	Perineum, female
Approach:	0	Open
Device:	Z	No device
Qualifier:	Z	No qualifier

FIGURE 4.5

0WQ

Section	0 Medical and Surgical
Body System	W Anatomical Regions, General
Operation	Q Repair: Restoring, to the extent possible, a body part to its normal anatomic structure and function

Body Part	Approach	Device	Qualifier
0 Head 2 Face 4 Upper Jaw 5 Lower Jaw 8 Chest Wall K Upper Back L Lower Back M Perineum, Male N Perineum, Female	0 Open 3 Percutaneous 4 Percutaneous Endoscopic X External	Z No Device	Z No Qualifier
6 Neck F Abdominal Wall	0 Open 3 Percutaneous 4 Percutaneous Endoscopic	Z No Device	Z No Qualifier
6 Neck F Abdominal Wall	X External	Z No Device	2 Stoma Z No Qualifier
C Mediastinum	0 Open 3 Percutaneous 4 Percutaneous Endoscopic	Z No Device	Z No Qualifier

Source: Adapted from ICD-10 Procedure Coding System (ICD-10-PCS) 2011 Tables and Index.

Access the ICD-10 Procedure Coding System (ICD-10-PCS) 2011 Tables and Index at www.cms.gov/ICD10/11b_2011_ICD10PCS.asp#TopOfPage.

Select 2011 Code Tables and Index.

Case Study 3

Correct answers:

3E0234Z

F13Z0ZZ

Rationale:

For the intramuscular hepatitis B vaccination, the ICD-10-PCS Index references all seven characters of the 3E0 root operation table:

Introduction

Muscle

Vaccine 3E0234Z

A review of the 3E0 root operation table and the operative report provides the information needed to verify the code:

Section:	3	Administration
Body system:	E	Physiological Systems and Anatomical Regions
Operation:	0	Introduction: Putting in or on a therapeutic, diagnostic, nutritional, physiological, or prophylactic substance except blood or blood products
Body system/region:	2	Muscle
Approach:	3	Percutaneous
Substance:	4	Serum, toxoid, and vaccine
Qualifier	Z	No qualifier

FIGURE 4.6

3E0

Section	**3**	Administration
Body System	**E**	Physiological Systems and Anatomical Regions
Operation	**0**	Introduction: Putting in or on a therapeutic, diagnostic, nutritional, physiological, or prophylactic substance except blood or blood products

Body System/Region	Approach	Device	Qualifier
0 Skin and Mucous Membranes	**X** External	**0** Antineoplastic	**5** Other Antineoplastic **M** Monoclonal Antibody
0 Skin and Mucous Membranes	**X** External	**2** Anti-infective	**8** Oxazolidinones **9** Other Anti-infective
0 Skin and Mucous Membranes	**X** External	**3** Anti-inflammatory **4** Serum, Toxoid and Vaccine **B** Local Anesthetic **K** Other Diagnostic Substance **M** Pigment **N** Analgesics, Hypnotics, Sedatives **T** Destructive Agent	**Z** No Qualifier
0 Skin and Mucous Membranes	**X** External	**G** Other Therapeutic Substance	**C** Other Substance
1 Subcutaneous Tissue	**3** Percutaneous	**0** Antineoplastic	**5** Other Antineoplastic **M** Monoclonal Antibody
1 Subcutaneous Tissue	**3** Percutaneous	**2** Anti-infective	**8** Oxazolidinones **9** Other Anti-infective
1 Subcutaneous Tissue	**3** Percutaneous	**3** Anti-inflammatory **4** Serum, Toxoid and Vaccine **6** Nutritional Substance **7** Electrolytic and Water Balance Substance **B** Local Anesthetic **H** Radioactive Substance **J** Contrast Agent **K** Other Diagnostic Substance **N** Analgesics, Hypnotics, Sedatives **T** Destructive Agent	**Z** No Qualifier

FIGURE
4.6

3E0 (cont.)

Body System/Region	Approach	Device	Qualifier
1 Subcutaneous Tissue	**3** Percutaneous	**G** Other Therapeutic Substance	**C** Other Substance
1 Subcutaneous Tissue	**3** Percutaneous	**V** Hormone	**G** Insulin **J** Other Hormone
2 Muscle	**3** Percutaneous	**0** Antineoplastic	**5** Other Antineoplastic **M** Monoclonal Antibody
2 Muscle	**3** Percutaneous	**2** Anti-infective	**8** Oxazolidinones **9** Other Anti-infective
2 Muscle	**3** Percutaneous	**3** Anti-inflammatory **4** Serum, Toxoid and Vaccine **6** Nutritional Substance **7** Electrolytic and Water Balance Substance **B** Local Anesthetic **H** Radioactive Substance **J** Contrast Agent **K** Other Diagnostic Substance **N** Analgesics, Hypnotics, Sedatives **T** Destructive Agent	**Z** No Qualifier
2 Muscle	**3** Percutaneous	**G** Other Therapeutic Substance	**C** Other Substance **N** Blood Brain Barrier Disruption
3 Peripheral Vein	**0** Open **3** Percutaneous	**0** Antineoplastic	**2** High-dose Interleukin-2 **3** Low-dose Interleukin-2 **5** Other Antineoplastic **M** Monoclonal Antibody **P** Clofarabine
3 Peripheral Vein	**0** Open **3** Percutaneous	**1** Thrombolytic	**6** Recombinant Human-activated Protein C **7** Other Thrombolytic
3 Peripheral Vein	**0** Open **3** Percutaneous	**2** Anti-infective	**8** Oxazolidinones **9** Other Anti-infective

FIGURE
4.6

3E0 (cont.)

Body System/Region	Approach	Device	Qualifier
3 Peripheral Vein	0 Open 3 Percutaneous	3 Anti-inflammatory 4 Serum, Toxoid and Vaccine 6 Nutritional Substance 7 Electrolytic and Water Balance Substance F Intracirculatory Anesthetic H Radioactive Substance J Contrast Agent K Other Diagnostic Substance N Analgesics, Hypnotics, Sedatives P Platelet Inhibitor R Antiarrhythmic T Destructive Agent X Vasopressor	Z No Qualifier
3 Peripheral Vein	0 Open 3 Percutaneous	G Other Therapeutic Substance	C Other Substance N Blood Brain Barrier Disruption
3 Peripheral Vein	0 Open 3 Percutaneous	U Pancreatic Islet Cells	0 Autologous 1 Nonautologous

Source: Adapted from ICD-10 Procedure Coding System (ICD-10-PCS) 2011 Tables and Index.

Access the ICD-10 Procedure Coding System (ICD-10-PCS) 2011 Tables and Index at www.cms.gov/ICD10/11b_2011_ICD10PCS.asp#TopOfPage.

Select 2011 Code Tables and Index.

Rationale:

For the newborn hearing screening, the ICD-10-PCS Index references the first four characters of the F13 root operation table:

Hearing assessment F13Z

A review of the F13 root operation table and the operative report provide the information needed to assign the remaining three characters of the code:

Section:	F	Physical rehabilitation and diagnostic audiology
Section qualifier:	1	Diagnostic audiology
Type:	3	Hearing assessment: measurement of hearing and related functions
Body system/region:	Z	None
Type qualifier:	0	Hearing screening
Equipment:	Z	None
Qualifier:	Z	None

FIGURE 4.7

F13

Section	**F** Physical Rehabilitation and Diagnostic Audiology
Body System	**1** Diagnostic Audiology
Operation	**3** Hearing Assessment: Measurement of hearing and related functions

Body System/Region	Type Qualifier	Equipment	Qualifier
Z None	**0** Hearing Screening	**0** Occupational Hearing **1** Audiometer **2** Sound Field/Booth **3** Tympanometer **8** Vestibular/Balance **9** Cochlear Implant **Z** None	**Z** None
Z None	**1** Pure Tone Audiometry, Air **2** Pure Tone Audiometry, Air and Bone	**0** Occupational Hearing **1** Audiometer **2** Sound Field/Booth **Z** None	**Z** None
Z None	**3** Bekesy Audiometry **6** Visual Reinforcement Audiometry **9** Short Increment Sensitivity Index **B** Stenger **C** Pure Tone Stenger	**1** Audiometer **2** Sound Field/Booth **Z** None	**Z** None
Z None	**4** Conditioned Play Audiometry **5** Select Picture Audiometry	**1** Audiometer **2** Sound Field/Booth **K** Audiovisual **Z** None	**Z** None
Z None	**7** Alternate Binaural or Monaural Loudness Balance	**1** Audiometer **K** Audiovisual **Z** None	**Z** None
Z None	**8** Tooth Decay **D** Tympanometry **F** Eustachian Tube Function **G** Acoustic Reflex Patterns **H** Acoustic Reflex Threshold **J** Acoustic Reflex Decay	**3** Tympanometer **4** Electroacoustic Immitance/ Acoustic Reflex **Z** None	**Z** None
Z None	**K** Electrocochleography **L** Auditory Evoked Potentials	**7** Electrophysiologic **Z** None	**Z** None

FIGURE
4.7

F13 (cont.)

Body System/Region	Type Qualifier	Equipment	Qualifier
Z None	M Evoked Otoacoustic Emissions, Screening N Evoked Otoacoustic Emissions, Diagnostic	6 Otoacoustic Emission (OAE) Z None	Z None
Z None	P Aural Rehabilitation Status	1 Audiometer 2 Sound Field/Booth 4 Electroacoustic Immitance/ Aucoustic Reflex 9 Cochlear Implant K Audiovisual L Assistive Listening P Computer	Z None
Z None	Q Auditory Processing	K Audiovisual P Computer Y Other Equipment Z None	Z None

Source: Adapted from ICD-10 Procedure Coding System (ICD-10-PCS) 2011 Tables and Index.

Access the ICD-10 Procedure Coding System (ICD-10-PCS) 2011 Tables and Index at www.cms.gov/ICD10/11b_2011_ICD10PCS.asp#TopOfPage.

Select 2011 Code Tables and Index.

Case Study 4

Correct answer:

10D00Z1

Rationale:

For the low segment transverse cesarean section, the ICD-10-PCS Index references the first four characters of the 10D root operation table:

Cesarean section *see* Extraction, Products of Conception 10D0

A review of the 10D root operation table and the operative report provides the information needed to assign the remaining three characters of the code:

Section:	1	Obstetrics
Body system:	0	Pregnancy
Operation:	D	Extraction: pulling or stripping out or off all or a portion of a body part
Body part:	0	Products of conception
Approach:	0	Open (uterine incision was performed)
Device:	Z	None
Qualifier:	1	Low cervical (low segment transverse incision was made)

FIGURE 4.8

10D

Section	**1** Obstetrics
Body System	**0** Pregnancy
Operation	**D** Extraction: Pulling or stripping out or off all or a portion of a body part

Body Part	Approach	Device	Qualifier
0 Products of Conception	**0** Open	**Z** No Device	**0** Classical **1** Low Cervical **2** Extraperitoneal
0 Products of Conception	**7** Via Natural or Artificial Opening	**Z** No Device	**3** Low Forceps **4** Mid Forceps **5** High Forceps **6** Vacuum **7** Internal Version **8** Other
1 Products of Conception, Retained **2** Products of Conception, Ectopic	**7** Via Natural or Artificial Opening **8** Via Natural or Artificial Opening, Endoscopic	**Z** No Device	**Z** No Qualifier

Source: Adapted from ICD-10 Procedure Coding System (ICD-10-PCS) 2011 Tables and Index.

Access the ICD-10 Procedure Coding System (ICD-10-PCS) 2011 Tables and Index at www.cms.gov/ICD10/11b_2011_ ICD10PCS.asp#TopOfPage.

Select 2011 Code Tables and Index.

Case Study 5

Correct answer:

0Y6M0ZD

0L8N3ZZ

Rationale:

A code is assigned for the transmetatarsal amputation and the percutaneous Achilles tendon lengthening. *ICD-10-PCS Coding Guidelines 2011*, guideline B3.2 states:

> *During the same operative episode, multiple procedures are coded if: … Multiple root operations with distinct objectives are performed on the same body part.*

The ICD-10-PCS Index references the first six characters of the 0Y6 root operation table for the right fourth toe transmetatarsal amputation:

Amputation *see* Detachment

Detachment

    Foot

        Right 0Y6M0Z

A review of the 0Y6 root operation table and the operative report provide the information needed to assign the remaining one character of the code:

Section:	0	Medical and Surgical
Body System:	Y	Anatomical Regions, Lower Extremities
Operation:	6	Detachment: Cutting off all or a portion of the upper or lower extremities
Body Part:	M	Foot, Right
Approach:	0	Open
Device:	Z	No Device
Qualifier:	D	Partial 4th Ray*

*Source: The *ICD-10-PCS Reference Manual 2011*, p. 2.13 states:

> Partial: Amputation anywhere along the shaft or head of the metacarpal bone of the hand, or of the metatarsal bone of the foot.

FIGURE 4.9

0Y6

Section	0	Medical and Surgical
Body System	Y	Anatomical Regions, Lower Extremities
Operation	6	Detachment: Cutting off all or a portion of the upper or lower extremities

Body System/Region	Type Qualifier	Equipment	Qualifier
2 Hindquarter, Right 3 Hindquarter, Left 4 Hindquarter, Bilateral 7 Femoral Region, Right 8 Femoral Region, Left F Knee Region, Right G Knee Region, Left	0 Open	Z No Device	Z No Qualifier
C Upper Leg, Right D Upper Leg, Left H Lower Leg, Right J Lower Leg, Left	0 Open	Z No Device	1 High 2 Mid 3 Low
M Foot, Right N Foot, Left	0 Open	Z No Device	0 Complete 4 Complete 1st Ray 5 Complete 2nd Ray 6 Complete 3rd Ray 7 Complete 4th Ray 8 Complete 5th Ray 9 Partial 1st Ray B Partial 2nd Ray C Partial 3rd Ray D Partial 4th Ray F Partial 5th Ray
P 1st Toe, Right Q 1st Toe, Left R 2nd Toe, Right S 2nd Toe, Left T 3rd Toe, Right U 3rd Toe, Left V 4th Toe, Right W 4th Toe, Left X 5th Toe, Right Y 5th Toe, Left	0 Open	Z No Device	0 Complete 1 High 2 Mid 3 Low

Source: Adapted from ICD-10 Procedure Coding System (ICD-10-PCS) 2011 Tables and Index.

Access the ICD-10 Procedure Coding System (ICD-10-PCS) 2011 Tables and Index at www.cms.gov/ICD10/11b_2011_ICD10PCS.asp#TopOfPage.

Select 2011 Code Tables and Index.

The ICD-10-PCS Index references the first three characters of the 0L8 root operation table for the right percutaneous Achilles tendon lengthening:

Lengthening

Tendon, by incision *see* Division, Tendons 0L8

A review of the 0L8 root operation table and the operative report provides the information needed to assign the remaining four characters of the code:

Section:	0	Medical and Surgical
Body system:	L	Tendons
Operation:	8	Division: Cutting into a body part, without draining fluids and/or gases from the body part, in order to separate or transect a body part
Body Part:	N	Lower Leg Tendon, Right*
Approach:	3	Percutaneous (stab incisions were made in the skin)
Device:	Z	No Device
Qualifier:	Z	No Qualifier

*"Definitions, Medical and Surgical–Body Part," *ICD-10-CM PCS Code Tables and Index 2011*, PDF file, p. 1095, states:

Lower Leg Tendon, Left and Lower Leg Tendon, Right – Includes: Achilles tendon.

FIGURE 4.10

0L8

Section	**0** Medical and Surgical
Body System	**L** Tendons
Operation	**8** Division: Cutting into a body part without draining fluids and/or gases from the body part in order to separate or transect a body part

Body System/Region	Type Qualifier	Equipment	Qualifier
0 Head and Neck Tendon **1** Shoulder Tendon, Right **2** Shoulder Tendon, Left **3** Upper Arm Tendon, Right **4** Upper Arm Tendon, Left **5** Lower Arm Tendon, Right **6** Lower Arm Tendon, Left **7** Hand Tendon, Right **8** Hand Tendon, Left **9** Trunk Tendon, Right **B** Trunk Tendon, Left **C** Thorax Tendon, Right **D** Thorax Tendon, Left **F** Abdomen Tendon, Right **G** Abdomen Tendon, Left **H** Perineum Tendon **J** Hip Tendon, Right **K** Hip Tendon, Left **L** Upper Leg Tendon, Right **M** Upper Leg Tendon, Left **N** Lower Leg Tendon, Right **P** Lower Leg Tendon, Left **Q** Knee Tendon, Right **R** Knee Tendon, Left **S** Ankle Tendon, Right **T** Ankle Tendon, Left **V** Foot Tendon, Right **W** Foot Tendon, Left	**0** Open **3** Percutaneous **4** Percutaneous Endoscopic	**Z** No Device	**Z** No Qualifier

Source: Adapted from ICD-10 Procedure Coding System (ICD-10-PCS) 2011 Tables and Index.

Access the ICD-10 Procedure Coding System (ICD-10-PCS) 2011 Tables and Index at www.cms.gov/ICD10/11b_2011_ICD10PCS.asp#TopOfPage.

Select 2011 Code Tables and Index.

Case Study 6

Correct answer:

0GTG0ZZ

0GTH0ZZ

07B10ZX

0CJS8ZZ

Rationale:

A code is assigned for the total thyroidectomy, the jugular lymph node biopsy, and the fiberoptic laryngoscopy.

ICD-10-PCS Coding Guidelines 2011, guideline B3.2, states:

> *During the same operative episode, multiple procedures are coded if...Multiple root operations with distinct objectives are performed on the same body part.*

The ICD-10-PCS Index references the first three characters of the 0GB and 0GT root operation tables for the total thyroidectomy:

Thyroidectomy

see Excision, Endocrine System 0GB

see Resection, Endocrine System 0GT

A review of the operative and pathology reports confirms that the entire thyroid was removed (both the left and right thyroid lobes), so this procedure is a resection. The root operation table 0GT provides the information needed to assign the remaining four characters of the code; however, two codes will be needed (one for each thyroid lobe that was removed):

Section:	0	Medical and surgical
Body system:	G	Endocrine system
Operation:	T	Resection: cutting out or off, without replacement, all of a body part
Body part:	G	Thyroid gland lobe, left
Approach:	0	Open
Device:	Z	No device
Qualifier:	Z	No qualifier

Section:	0	Medical and surgical
Body system:	G	Endocrine system
Operation:	T	Resection: cutting out or off, without replacement, all of a body part
Body part:	H	Thyroid gland lobe, right
Approach:	0	Open
Device:	Z	No device
Qualifier:	Z	No qualifier

FIGURE 4.11   **0GT**

Section	**0** Medical and Surgical		
Body System	**G** Endocrine System		
Operation	**T** Resection: Cutting out or off, without replacement, all of a body part		

Body Part	*Approach*	*Device*	*Qualifier*
0 Pituitary Gland **1** Pineal Body **2** Adrenal Gland, Left **3** Adrenal Gland, Right **4** Adrenal Glands, Bilateral **6** Carotid Body, Left **7** Carotid Body, Right **8** Carotid Bodies, Bilateral **9** Para-aortic Body **B** Coccygeal Glomus **C** Glomus Jugulare **D** Aortic Body **F** Paraganglion Extremity **G** Thyroid Gland Lobe, Left **H** Thyroid Gland Lobe, Right **K** Thyroid Gland **L** Superior Parathyroid Gland, Right **M** Superior Parathyroid Gland, Left **N** Inferior Parathyroid Gland, Right **P** Inferior Parathyroid Gland, Left **Q** Parathyroid Glands, Multiple **R** Parathyroid Gland	**0** Open **4** Percutaneous Endoscopic	**Z** No Device	**Z** No Qualifier

Source: Adapted from ICD-10 Procedure Coding System (ICD-10-PCS) 2011 Tables and Index.

Access the ICD-10 Procedure Coding System (ICD-10-PCS) 2011 Tables and Index at www.cms.gov/ICD10/11b_2011_ICD10PCS.asp#TopOfPage.

Select 2011 Code Tables and Index.

For the right jugular lymph node biopsy, the ICD-10-PCS Index references the first four characters of the 07B root operation table:

Biopsy

see Excision, Diagnostic

Excision

    Lymphatic

       Neck*

          Right 07B1

*"Definitions, Medical and Surgical–Body Part," *ICD-10-CM PCS Code Tables and Index 2011* PDF file, p. 1098, states:

Lymphatic, Right Neck–Includes: Jugular lymph node.

A review of the 07B root operation table and the operative report provides the information needed to assign the remaining three characters of the code:

Section:	0	Medical and surgical
Body system:	7	Lymphatic and hemic systems
Operation:	B	Excision: cutting out or off, without replacement, a portion of a body part
Body part:	1	Lymphatic, right neck
Approach:	0	Open (the node was dissected free)
Device:	Z	No device
Qualifier:	X	Diagnostic (the ICD-10-PCS Index states for "Biopsy, see Excision, Diagnostic")

FIGURE 4.12   **07B**

Section	**0** Medical and Surgical
Body System	**7** Lymphatic and Hemic Systems
Operation	**B** Excision: Cutting out or off, without replacement, a portion of a body part

Body Part	Approach	Device	Qualifier
0 Lymphatic, Head **1** Lymphatic, Right Neck **2** Lymphatic, Left Neck **3** Lymphatic, Right Upper Extremity **4** Lymphatic, Left Upper Extremity **5** Lymphatic, Right Axillary **6** Lymphatic, Left Axillary **7** Lymphatic, Thorax **8** Lymphatic, Internal Mammary, Right **9** Lymphatic, Internal Mammary, Left **B** Lymphatic, Mesenteric **C** Lymphatic, Pelvis **D** Lymphatic, Aortic **F** Lymphatic, Right Lower Extremity **G** Lymphatic, Left Lower Extremity **H** Lymphatic, Right Inguinal **J** Lymphatic, Left Inguinal **K** Thoracic Duct **L** Cisterna Chyli **M** Thymus **P** Spleen	**0** Open **3** Percutaneous **4** Percutaneous Endoscopic	**Z** No Device	**X** Diagnostic **Z** No Qualifier

Source: Adapted from ICD-10 Procedure Coding System (ICD-10-PCS) 2011 Tables and Index.

Access the ICD-10 Procedure Coding System (ICD-10-PCS) 2011 Tables and Index at www.cms.gov/ICD10/11b_2011_ICD10PCS.asp#TopOfPage.

Select 2011 Code Tables and Index.

The ICD-10-PCS Index references all seven characters of the 0CJ root operation table for the fiberoptic laryngoscopy:

Laryngoscopy 0CJS8ZZ

A review of the 0CJ root operation table and the operative report provides the information needed to verify the code:

Section:	0	Medical and surgical
Body system:	C	Mouth and throat
Operation:	J	Inspection: visually and/or manually exploring a body part
Body part:	S	Larynx
Approach:	8	Via natural or artificial opening endoscopic
Device:	Z	No device
Qualifier:	Z	No qualifier

FIGURE 4.13

0CJ

Section	0 Medical and Surgical
Body System	C Mouth and Throat
Operation	J Inspection: Visually and/or manually exploring a body part

Body Part	Approach	Device	Qualifier
A Salivary Gland	**0** Open **3** Percutaneous **X** External	**Z** No Device	**Z** No Qualifier
S Larynx **Y** Mouth and Throat	**0** Open **3** Percutaneous **4** Percutaneous Endoscopic **7** Via Natural or Artificial Opening **8** Via Natural or Artificial Opening Endoscopic **X** External	**Z** No Device	**Z** No Qualifier

Source: Adapted from ICD-10 Procedure Coding System (ICD-10-PCS) 2011 Tables and Index.

Access the ICD-10 Procedure Coding System (ICD-10-PCS) 2011 Tables and Index at www.cms.gov/ICD10/11b_2011_ICD10PCS.asp#TopOfPage.

Select 2011 Code Tables and Index.

Case Study 7

Correct answer:

0QS604Z

30233N1

Rationale:

A code is assigned for the open reduction with internal fixation of proximal femur fracture and for the blood transfusion.

ICD-10-PCS Coding Guidelines 2011, guideline B3.2, states:

> *During the same operative episode, multiple procedures are coded if … Multiple root operations with distinct objectives are performed on the same body part.*

The ICD-10-PCS Index references the first four characters of the 0QS root operation table for the open reduction, internal fixation of the right proximal femur with bone graft and multiple cerclage cables and Zimmer® Cable-Ready® plate:

Reduction

Fracture *see* Reposition

Reposition

　Femur

　　Upper*

　　　Right 0QS6

*The proximal part of the femur is the part that is close to pelvis. (The distal part of the femur is close to the knee).

A review of the 0QS root operation table and the operative report provides the information needed to assign the remaining three characters of the code:

Section:	0	Medical and surgical
Body system:	Q	Lower bones
Operation:	S	Reposition: moving to its normal location, or other suitable location, all or a portion of a body part
Body part:	6	Upper femur, right
Approach:	0	Open (an incision was made through the femur)
Device:	4	Internal fixation (cerclage cables, pin, plate, bone graft)
Qualifier:	Z	No qualifier

FIGURE 4.14

0QS

Section	0	Medical and Surgical
Body System	Q	Lower Bones
Operation	S	Reposition: Moving to its normal location, or other suitable location, all or a portion of a body part

Body Part	Approach	Device	Qualifier
0 Lumbar Vertebra **1** Sacrum **4** Acetabulum, Right **5** Acetabulum, Left **S** Coccyx	**0** Open **3** Percutaneous **4** Percutaneous Endoscopic	**4** Internal Fixation Device **Z** No Device	**Z** No Qualifier
0 Lumbar Vertebra **1** Sacrum **4** Acetabulum, Right **5** Acetabulum, Left **S** Coccyx	**X** External	**Z** No Device	**Z** No Qualifier

FIGURE 4.14

Body Part	Approach	Device	Qualifier
2 Pelvic Bone, Right **3** Pelvic Bone, Left **D** Patella, Right **F** Patella, Left **L** Tarsal, Right **M** Tarsal, Left **N** Metatarsal, Right **P** Metatarsal, Left **Q** Toe Phalanx, Right **R** Toe Phalanx, Left	**0** Open **3** Percutaneous **4** Percutaneous Endoscopic	**4** Internal Fixation Device **Z** No Device	**Z** No Qualifier
2 Pelvic Bone, Right **3** Pelvic Bone, Left **D** Patella, Right **F** Patella, Left **L** Tarsal, Right **M** Tarsal, Left **N** Metatarsal, Right **P** Metatarsal, Left **Q** Toe Phalanx, Right **R** Toe Phalanx, Left	**0** Open **3** Percutaneous **4** Percutaneous Endoscopic	**5** External Fixation Device	**3** Monoplanar **4** Ring **5** Hybrid **Z** No Qualifier
2 Pelvic Bone, Right **3** Pelvic Bone, Left **D** Patella, Right **F** Patella, Left **L** Tarsal, Right **M** Tarsal, Left **N** Metatarsal, Right **P** Metatarsal, Left **Q** Toe Phalanx, Right **R** Toe Phalanx, Left	**X** External	**Z** No Device	**Z** No Qualifier

FIGURE 4.14

0QS (cont.)

Body Part	Approach	Device	Qualifier
6 Upper Femur, Right **7** Upper Femur, Left **8** Femoral Shaft, Right **9** Femoral Shaft, Left **B** Lower Femur, Right **C** Lower Femur, Left **G** Tibia, Right **H** Tibia, Left **J** Fibula, Right **K** Fibula, Left	**0** Open **3** Percutaneous **4** Percutaneous Endoscopic	**4** Internal Fixation Device **6** Intramedullary Fixation Device **Z** No Device	**Z** No Qualifier
6 Upper Femur, Right **7** Upper Femur, Left **8** Femoral Shaft, Right **9** Femoral Shaft, Left **B** Lower Femur, Right **C** Lower Femur, Left **G** Tibia, Right **H** Tibia, Left **J** Fibula, Right **K** Fibula, Left	**0** Open **3** Percutaneous **4** Percutaneous Endoscopic	**5** External Fixation Device	**3** Monoplanar **4** Ring **5** Hybrid **Z** No Qualifier
6 Upper Femur, Right **7** Upper Femur, Left **8** Femoral Shaft, Right **9** Femoral Shaft, Left **B** Lower Femur, Right **C** Lower Femur, Left **G** Tibia, Right **H** Tibia, Left **J** Fibula, Right **K** Fibula, Left	**X** External	**Z** No Device	**Z** No Qualifier

Source: Adapted from ICD-10 Procedure Coding System (ICD-10-PCS) 2011 Tables and Index.

Access the ICD-10 Procedure Coding System (ICD-10-PCS) 2011 Tables and Index at www.cms.gov/ICD10/11b_2011_ICD10PCS.asp#TopOfPage.

Select 2011 Code Tables and Index.

The ICD-10-PCS Index references the first four characters of the 302 root operation table for the intraoperative transfusion of two units of packed red blood cells:

Transfusion

    Vein

        Peripheral

            Blood

                Red Cells 3023

A review of the 302 root operation table and the operative report provides the information needed to assign the remaining three characters of the code:

Section:	3	Administration
Body system:	0	Circulatory
Operation:	2	Transfusion: putting in blood or blood products
Body system/region:	3	Peripheral vein
Approach:	3	Percutaneous
Substance:	N	Red blood cells
Qualifier:	1	Nonautologous (the source of the blood was the blood bank)

FIGURE 4.15

302

Section	**3**	Administration
Body System	**0**	Circulatory
Operation	**2**	Transfusion: Putting in blood or blood products

Body System/Region	Approach	Substance	Qualifier
3 Peripheral Vein **4** Central Vein	**0** Open **3** Percutaneous	**A** Stem Cells, Embryonic	**Z** No Qualifier
3 Peripheral Vein **4** Central Vein	**0** Open **3** Percutaneous	**G** Bone Marrow **H** Whole Blood **J** Serum Albumin **K** Frozen Plasma **L** Fresh Plasma **M** Plasma Cryoprecipitate **N** Red Blood Cells **P** Frozen Red Cells **Q** White Cells **R** Platelets **S** Globulin **T** Fibrinogen **V** Antihemophilic Factors **W** Factor IX **X** Stem Cells, Cord Blood **Y** Stem Cells, Hematopoietic	**0** Autologous **1** Nonautologous
5 Peripheral Artery **6** Central Artery	**0** Open **3** Percutaneous	**G** Bone Marrow **H** Whole Blood **J** Serum Albumin **K** Frozen Plasma **L** Fresh Plasma **M** Plasma Cryoprecipitate **N** Red Blood Cells **P** Frozen Red Cells **Q** White Cells **R** Platelets **S** Globulin **T** Fibrinogen **V** Antihemophilic Factors **W** Factor IX **X** Stem Cells, Cord Blood **Y** Stem Cells, Hematopoietic	**0** Autologous **1** Nonautologous

FIGURE 4.15

302 (cont.)

Body System/Region	Approach	Substance	Qualifier
7 Products of Conception, Circulatory	**3** Percutaneous **7** Via natural or Artificial Opening	**H** Whole Blood **J** Serum Albumin **K** Frozen Plasma **L** Fresh Plasma **M** Plasma Cryoprecipitate **N** Red Blood Cells **P** Frozen Red Cells **Q** White Cells **R** Platelets **S** Globulin **T** Fibrinogen **V** Antihemophilic Factors **W** Factor IX	**1** Nonautologous

Source: Adapted from ICD-10 Procedure Coding System (ICD-10-PCS) 2011 Tables and Index.

Access the ICD-10 Procedure Coding System (ICD-10-PCS) 2011 Tables and Index at www.cms.gov/ICD10/11b_2011_ICD10PCS.asp#TopOfPage.

Select 2011 Code Tables and Index.

Case Study 8

Correct answer:

0SRD0JZ

Rationale:

The ICD-10-PCS Index references the first five characters of the 0SR root operation table for the left total knee replacement:

Replacement

Joint

Knee Left 0SRD0

A review of the 0SR root operation table and the operative report provides the information needed to assign the remaining two characters of the code:

Section:	0	Medical and surgical
Body system:	S	Lower joints
Operation:	R	Replacement: putting in or on biological or synthetic material that physically takes the place and/or function of all or a portion of a body part
Body part:	D	Knee joint, left
Approach:	0	Open
Device:	J	Synthetic substitute (the prosthetics were made of polyethylene)
Qualifier:	Z	No qualifier

FIGURE 4.16

0SR

Section	**0**	Medical and Surgical
Body System	**S**	Lower Joints
Operation	**R**	Replacement: Putting in or on biological or synthetic material that physically takes the place and/or function of all or a portion of a body part

Body Part	Approach	Device	Qualifier
0 Lumbar Vertebral Joint **3** Lumbosacral Joint	**0** Open	**7** Autologous Tissue Substitute **K** nonautologous Tissue Substitute	**Z** No Qualifier
0 Lumbar Vertebral Joint **3** Lumbosacral Joint	**0** Open	**J** Synthetic Substitute	**4** Facet **Z** No Qualifier
2 Lumbar Vertebral Disc **4** Lumbosacral Disc **5** Sacrococcygeal Joint **6** Coccygeal Joint **7** Sacroiliac Joint, Right **8** Sacroiliac Joint, Left **C** Knee Joint, Right **D** Knee Joint, Left **F** Ankle Joint, Right **G** Ankle Joint, Left **H** Tarsal Joint, Right **J** Tarsal Joint, Left **K** Metatarsal-Tarsal Joint, Right **L** Metatarsal-Tarsal Joint, Left **M** Metatarsal-Phalangeal Joint, Right **N** Metatarsal-Phalangeal Joint, Left **P** Toe Phalangeal Joint, Right **Q** Toe Phalangeal Joint, Left **T** Knee Joint, Femoral Surface, Right **U** Knee Joint, Femoral Surface, Left **V** Knee Joint, Tibial Surface, Right **W** Knee Joint, Tibial Surface, Left	**0** Open	**7** Autologous Tissue Substitute **J** Synthetic Substitute **K** Nonautologous Tissue Substitute	**Z** No Qualifier
9 Hip Joint, Right **B** Hip Joint, Left	**0** Open	**7** Autologous Tissue Substitute **K** Nonautologous Tissue Substitute	**Z** No Qualifier

---

FIGURE 4.16

0SR (cont.)

Body Part	Approach	Device	Qualifier
9 Hip Joint, Right **B** Hip Joint, Left	**0** Open	**J** Synthetic Substitute	**5** Metal on Polyethylene **6** Metal on Metal **7** Ceramic on Ceramic **8** Ceramic on Polyethylene **Z** No Qualifier
A Hip Joint, Acetabular Surface, Right **E** Hip Joint, Acetabular Surface, Left	**0** Open	**7** Autologous Tissue Substitute **K** Nonautologous Tissue Substitute	**Z** No Qualifier

Source: Adapted from ICD-10 Procedure Coding System (ICD-10-PCS) 2011 Tables and Index.

Access the ICD-10 Procedure Coding System (ICD-10-PCS) 2011 Tables and Index at www.cms.gov/ICD10/11b_2011_ICD10PCS.asp#TopOfPage.

Select 2011 Code Tables and Index.

Case Study 9

Correct answer:

0SPD0JZ

0SHD08Z

Rationale:

A code is assigned for the removal of the left total knee replacement and for the insertion of the methylmethacrylate spacers.

ICD-10-PCS Coding Guidelines 2011, guideline B3.2, states:

> *During the same operative episode, multiple procedures are coded if... Multiple root operations with distinct objectives are performed on the same body part.*

The ICD-10-PCS Index references the first four characters of the 0SP root operation table for removal of the left total knee replacement:

Removal of device from*

Joint

Knee

Left 0SPD

*ICD-10-PCS Reference Manual 2011, p. 2.51, states:

A removal procedure is coded for taking out the device used in a previous replacement procedure.

A review of the 0SP root operation table and the operative report provides the information needed to assign the remaining three characters of the code:

Section:	0	Medical and surgical
Body system:	S	Lower joints
Operation:	P	Removal: taking out or off a device from a body part
Body part:	D	Knee joint, left
Approach:	0	Open
Device:	J	Synthetic substitute (prosthetic femoral and tibial components were removed)
Qualifier:	Z	No qualifier

FIGURE 4.17

0SP

Section	0	Medical and Surgical
Body System	S	Lower Joints
Operation	P	Removal: Taking out or off a device from a body part

Body Part	Approach	Device	Qualifier
0 Lumbar Vertebral Joint **3** Lumbosacral Joint **5** Sacrococcygeal Joint **6** Coccygeal Joint **7** Sacroiliac Joint, Right **8** Sacroiliac Joint, Left	**0** Open **3** Percutaneous **4** Percutaneous Endoscopic	**0** Drainage Device **3** Infusion Device **4** Internal Fixation Device **7** Autologous Tissue Substitute **8** Spacer **J** Synthetic Substitute **K** Nonautologous Tissue Substitute	**Z** No Qualifier
0 Lumbar Vertebral Joint **3** Lumbosacral Joint **5** Sacrococcygeal Joint **6** Coccygeal Joint **7** Sacroiliac Joint, Right **8** Sacroiliac Joint, Left	**X** External	**0** Drainage Device **3** Infusion Device **4** Internal Fixation Device	**Z** No Qualifier
2 Lumbosacral Vertebral Disc **4** Lumbosacral Disc	**0** Open **3** Percutaneous **4** Percutaneous Endoscopic	**0** Drainage Device **3** Infusion Device **7** Autologous Tissue Substitute **J** Synthetic Substitute **K** Nonautologous Tissue Substitute	**Z** No Qualifier
2 Lumbosacral Vertebral Disc **4** Lumbosacral Disc	**X** External	**0** Drainage Device **3** Infusion Device	**Z** No Qualifier
9 Hip Joint, Right **B** Hip joint, Left	**0** Open	**0** Drainage Device **3** Infusion Device **4** Internal Fixation Device **5** External Fixation Device **7** Autologous Tissue Substitute **8** Spacer **9** Liner **B** Resurfacing Device **J** Synthetic Substitute **K** Nonautologous Tissue Substitute	**Z** No Qualifier

FIGURE 4.17

0SP (cont.)

Body Part	Approach	Device	Qualifier
9 Hip Joint, Right **B** Hip Joint, Left	**3** Percutaneous **4** Percutaneous Endoscopic	**0** Drainage Device **3** Infusion Device **4** Internal Fixation Device **5** External Fixation Device **7** Autologous Tissue Substitute **8** Spacer **J** Synthetic Substitute **K** Nonautologous Tissue Substitute	**Z** No Qualifier
9 Hip Joint, Right **B** Hip Joint, Left	**X** External	**0** Drainage Device **3** Infusion Device **4** Internal Fixation Device **5** External Fixation Device	**Z** No Qualifier
C Knee Joint, Right **D** Knee Joint, Left	**0** Open	**0** Drainage Device **3** Infusion Device **4** Internal Fixation Device **5** External Fixation Device **7** Autologous Tissue Substitute **8** Spacer **9** Liner **J** Synthetic Substitute **K** Nonautologous Tissue Substitute	**Z** No Qualifier
C Knee Joint, Right **D** Knee Joint, Left	**3** Percutaneous **4** Percutaneous Endoscopic	**0** Drainage Device **3** Infusion Device **4** Internal Fixation Device **5** External Fixation Device **7** Autologous Tissue Substitute **8** Spacer **9** Liner **J** Synthetic Substitute **K** Nonautologous Tissue Substitute	**Z** No Qualifier
C Knee Joint, Right **D** Knee Joint, Left	**X** External	**0** Drainage Device **3** Infusion Device **4** Internal Fixation Device **5** External Fixation Device	**Z** No Qualifier

FIGURE 4.17

0SP (cont.)

Body Part	Approach	Device	Qualifier
F Ankle Fracture, Right **G** Ankle Fracture, Left **H** Tarsal Joint, Right **J** Tarsal Joint, Left **K** Metatarsal-Tarsal Joint, Right **L** Metatarsal-Tarsal Joint, Left **M** Metatarsal-Phalangeal Joint, Right **N** Metatarsal-Phalangeal Joint, Left **P** Toe Phalangeal Joint, Right **Q** Toe Phalangeal Joint, Left	**0** Open **3** Percutaneous **4** Percutaneous Endoscopic	**0** Drainage Device **3** Infusion Device **4** Internal Fixation Device **5** External Fixation Device **7** Autologous Tissue Substitute **8** Spacer **J** Synthetic Substitute **K** Nonautologous Tissue Substitute	**Z** No Qualifier
F Ankle Fracture, Right **G** Ankle Fracture, Left **H** Tarsal Joint, Right **J** Tarsal Joint, Left **K** Metatarsal-Tarsal Joint, Right **L** Metatarsal-Tarsal Joint, Left **M** Metatarsal-Phalangeal Joint, Right **N** Metatarsal-Phalangeal Joint, Left **P** Toe Phalangeal Joint, Right **Q** Toe Phalangeal Joint, Left	**X** External	**0** Drainage Device **3** Infusion Device **4** Internal Fixation Device **5** External Fixation Device	**Z** No Qualifier

Source: Adapted from ICD-10 Procedure Coding System (ICD-10-PCS) 2011 Tables and Index.

Access the ICD-10 Procedure Coding System (ICD-10-PCS) 2011 Tables and Index at www.cms.gov/ICD10/11b_2011_ICD10PCS.asp#TopOfPage.

Select 2011 Code Tables and Index.

The ICD-10-PCS Index references the first four characters of the 0SH root operation table for the insertion of methylmethacrylate spacers into the left knee:

Insertion of device in

Joint

Knee

Left 0SHD

A review of the 0SH root operation table and the operative report provides the information needed to assign the remaining three characters of the code:

Section:	0	Medical and surgical
Body system:	S	Lower joints
Operation:	H	Insertion: putting in a nonbiological appliance that monitors, assists, performs, or prevents a physiological function but does not physically take the place of a body part
Body part:	D	Knee joint, left
Approach:	0	Open
Device:	8	Spacer
Qualifier:	Z	No qualifier

FIGURE 4.18

0SH

Section	**0**	Medical and Surgical
Body System	**S**	Lower Joints
Operation	**H**	Insertion: Putting in a nonbiological appliance that monitors, assists, performs, or prevents a physiological function but does not physically take the place of a body part

Body Part	Approach	Device	Qualifier
0 Lumbar Vertebral Joint **3** Lumbosacral Joint	**0** Open **3** Percutaneous **4** Percutaneous Endoscopic	**3** Infusion Device **8** Spacer	**Z** No Qualifier
0 Lumbar Vertebral Joint **3** Lumbosacral Joint	**0** Open **3** Percutaneous **4** Percutaneous Endoscopic	**4** Internal Fixation Device	**2** Interspinous Process **3** Pedicle-based Dynamic Stabilization **Z** No Qualifier
1 Lumbar Vertebral Disc **4** Lumbosacral Disc	**0** Open **3** Percutaneous **4** Percutaneous Endoscopic	**3** Infusion Device **8** Spacer	**Z** No Qualifier
5 Sacrococcygeal Joint **6** Coccygeal Joint **7** Sacroiliac Joint, Right **8** Sacroiliac Joint, Left	**0** Open **3** Percutaneous **4** Percutaneous Endoscopic	**3** Infusion Device **4** Internal Fixation Device **8** Spacer	**Z** No Qualifier
9 Hip Joint, Right **B** Hip Joint, Left **C** Knee Joint, Right **D** Knee Joint, Left **F** Ankle Joint, Right **G** Ankle Joint, Left **H** Tarsal Joint, Right **J** Tarsal Joint, Left **K** Metatarsal-Tarsal Joint, Right **L** Metatarsal-Tarsal Joint, Left **M** Metatarsal-Phalangeal Joint, Right **N** Metatarsal-Phalangeal Joint, Left **P** Toe Phalangeal Joint, Right **Q** Toe Phalangeal Joint, Left	**0** Open **3** Percutaneous **4** Percutaneous Endoscopic	**3** Infusion Device **4** Internal Fixation Device **5** External Fixation Device **8** Spacer	**Z** No Qualifier

Source: Adapted from ICD-10 Procedure Coding System (ICD-10-PCS) 2011 Tables and Index.

Access the ICD-10 Procedure Coding System (ICD-10-PCS) 2011 Tables and Index at www.cms.gov/ICD10/11b_2011_ICD10PCS.asp#TopOfPage.

Select 2011 Code Tables and Index.

Case Study 10

Correct answer:

00160J6

Rationale:

ICD-10-PCS Coding Guidelines 2011, guideline B3.6a, states:

> *Bypass procedures are coded by identifying the body part bypassed "from" and the body part bypassed "to." The fourth character body part specifies the body part bypassed from, and the qualifier specifies the body part bypassed to.*

For the insertion of a ventriculoperitoneal shunt, the ICD-10-PCS Index references the first five characters of the 001 root operation table:

Shunt creation *see* Bypass

Bypass

Cerebral Ventricle 00160

A review of the 001 root operation table and the operative report provide the information needed to assign the remaining two characters of the code:

Section:	0	Medical and surgical
Body system:	0	Central nervous system
Operation:	1	Bypass: altering the route of passage of the contents of a tubular body part
Body part:	6	Cerebral ventricle
Approach:	0	Open
Device:	J	Synthetic substitute (programmable valve set)
Qualifier:	6	Peritoneal cavity

FIGURE 4.19

Section	**0**	Medical and Surgical
Body System	**0**	Central Nervous System
Operation	**1**	Bypass: Altering the route of passage of the contents of a tubular body part

Body Part	Approach	Device	Qualifier
6 Cerebral Ventricle	**0** Open	**7** Autologous Tissue Substitute **J** Synthetic Substitute **K** Nonautologous Tissue Substitute	**0** Nasopharynx **1** Mastoid Sinus **2** Atrium **3** Blood Vessel **4** Pleural Cavity **5** Intestine **6** Peritoneal Cavity **7** Urinary Tract **8** Bone Marrow **B** Cerebral Cisterns
U Spinal Canal	**0** Open	**7** Autologous Tissue Substitute **J** Synthetic Substitute **K** Nonautologous Tissue Substitute	**4** Pleural Cavity **6** Peritoneal Cavity **7** Urinary Tract **9** Fallopian Tube

Source: Adapted from ICD-10 Procedure Coding System (ICD-10-PCS) 2011 Tables and Index.

Access the ICD-10 Procedure Coding System (ICD-10-PCS) 2011 Tables and Index at www.cms.gov/ICD10/11b_2011_ICD10PCS.asp#TopOfPage.

Select 2011 Code Tables and Index.

Case Study 11

Correct answer:

0RG2040

Rationale:

For the C4-C5, C5-C6, and C6-C7 anterior cervical discectomy with fusion, placement of milled structural allograft and anterior cervical plating, the ICD-10-PCS Index references the first four characters of the 0RG root operation table:

Fusion

Cervical Vertebral

2 or more 0RG2

A review of the 0RG root operation table and the operative report provides the information needed to assign the remaining three characters of the code:

Section:	0	Medical and surgical
Body system:	R	Upper joints
Operation:	G	Fusion: joining together portions of an articular body part rendering the articular body part immobile
Body part:	2	Cervical vertebral joints, two or more (three joints were fused: C4-C5, C5-C6, and C6-C7)
Approach:	0	Open
Device:	4	Internal fixation device*
Qualifier:	0	Anterior approach, anterior column

*ICD-10-PCS Coding Guidelines 2011, guideline B3.10c, states:

Combinations of devices and materials are often used on a vertebral joint to render the joint immobile. When combinations of devices are used on the same vertebral joint, the device value coded for the procedure is as follows: ... if internal fixation is used to render the joint immobile and an interbody fusion device is not used, the procedure is coded with the device value Internal Fixation Device. ... Examples ... Fusion of a vertebral joint using rigid plates affixed with screws and reinforced with bone cement is coded to the device Internal Fixation Device.

FIGURE 4.20

0RG

Section	0	Medical and Surgical
Body System	R	Upper Joints
Operation	G	Fusion: Joining together portions of an articular body part rendering the body part immobile

Body Part	Approach	Device	Qualifier
0 Occipital-cervical Joint 1 Cervical Vertebral Joint 2 Cervical Vertebral Joints, 2 or more 4 Cervicothoracic Vertebral Joint 6 Thoracic Vertebral Joint 7 Thoracic Vertebral Joints, 2 to 7 8 Thoracic Vertebral Joints, 8 or more A Thoracolumbar Vertebral Joint	0 Open 3 Percutaneous 4 Percutaneous Endoscopic	3 Interbody Fusion Device 4 Internal Fixation Device 7 Autologous Tissue Substitute J Synthetic Substitute K Nonautologous Tissue Substitute Z No Device	0 Anterior Approach, Anterior Column 1 Posterior Approach, Posterior Column J Posterior Approach, Anterior Column
C Temporomandibular Joint, Right D Temporomandibular Joint, Left E Sternoclavicular Joint, Right F Sternoclavicular Joint, Left G Acromioclavicular Joint, Right H Acromioclavicular Joint, Left J Shoulder Joint, Right K Shoulder Joint, Left	0 Open 3 Percutaneous 4 Percutaneous Endoscopic	4 Internal Fixation Device 7 Autologous Tissue Substitute J Synthetic Substitute K Nonautologous Tissue Substitute Z No Device	Z No Qualifier
L Elbow Joint, Right M Elbow Joint, Left N Wrist Joint, Right P Wrist Joint, Left Q Carpal Joint, Right R Carpal Joint, Left S Metacarpocarpal Joint, Right T Metacarpocarpal Joint, Left U Metacarpophalangeal Joint, Right V Metacarpophalangeal Joint, Left W Finger Phalangeal Joint, Right X Finger Phalangeal Joint, Left	0 Open 3 Percutaneous 4 Percutaneous Endoscopic	4 Internal Fixation Device 5 External Fixation 7 Autologous Tissue Substitute J Synthetic Substitute K Nonautologous Tissue Substitute Z No Device	Z No Qualifier

Source: Adapted from ICD-10 Procedure Coding System (ICD-10-PCS) 2011 Tables and Index.

Access the ICD-10 Procedure Coding System (ICD-10-PCS) 2011 Tables and Index at www.cms.gov/ICD10/11b_2011_ICD10PCS.asp#TopOfPage.

Select 2011 Code Tables and Index.

Case Study 12

Correct answer:

0HHV0NZ

0KXH0ZZ

0KXJ0ZZ

Rationale:

For the bilateral breast placement of tissue expanders, the ICD-10-PCS Index references the first four characters of the 0HH root operation table:

Tissue Expander

    Insertion of device in

        Breast

            Bilateral 0HHV

A review of the 0HH root operation table and the operative report provides the information needed to assign the remaining three characters of the code:

Section:	0	Medical and surgical
Body system:	H	Skin and breast
Operation:	H	Insertion: putting in a nonbiological appliance that monitors, assists, performs, or prevents a physiological function but does not physically take the place of a body part
Body part:	V	Breast, bilateral
Approach:	0	Open
Device:	N	Tissue expander
Qualifier:	Z	No qualifier

FIGURE 4.21

0HH

Section	0	Medical and Surgical
Body System	H	Skin and Breast
Operation	H	Insertion: Putting in a nonbiological appliance that monitors, assists, performs, or prevents a physiological function but does not physically take the place of a body part

Body Part	Approach	Device	Qualifier
T Breast, Right **U** Breast, Left **V** Breast, Bilateral **W** Nipple, Right **X** Nipple, Left	**0** Open **3** Percutaneous **7** Via Natural or Artificial Opening **8** Via Natural or artificial Opening, Endoscopic	**1** Radioactive Element **N** Tissue Expander	**Z** No Qualifier
T Breast, Right **U** Breast, Left **V** Breast, Bilateral **W** Nipple, Right **X** Nipple, Left	**X** External	**1** Radioactive Element	**Z** No Qualifier

Source: Adapted from ICD-10 Procedure Coding System (ICD-10-PCS) 2011 Tables and Index.

Access the ICD-10 Procedure Coding System (ICD-10-PCS) 2011 Tables and Index at www.cms.gov/ICD10/11b_2011_ICD10PCS.asp#TopOfPage.

Select 2011 Code Tables and Index.

The ICD-10-PCS Index references the first four characters of the OKX root operation table for the bilateral serratus anterior muscle flap:

Serratus anterior muscle

use Muscle, Thorax, Left

use Muscle, Thorax, Right

Transfer

   Muscle

      Thorax

         Left 0KXJ

            Right 0KXH

A review of the 0KX root operation table and the operative report provides the information needed to assign the remaining three characters of each code—two codes are needed to classify the bilateral serratus anterior muscle flaps:

Section:	0	Medical and surgical
Body system:	K	Muscles
Operation:	X	Transfer: moving, without taking out, all or a portion of a body part to another location to take over the function of all or a portion of a body part
Body part:	J	Thorax muscle, left
Approach:	0	Open
Device:	Z	No device
Qualifier:	Z	No qualifier*

*The ICD-10-PCS Index references thorax muscles for a serratus anterior muscle transfer, so there is no other tissue to be reported with the qualifier.

ICD-10-PCS Reference Manual 2011, p. 2.35, states:

> *For the transfer root operation, the body system value describes the deepest tissue layer in the flap. The qualifier can be used to describe the other tissue layers, if any, being transferred.*

FIGURE 4.22

0KX

Section	**0** Medical and Surgical
Body System	**K** Muscles
Operation	**X** Transfer: Moving, without taking out, all or a portion of a body part to another location to take over the function of all or a portion of a body part

Body Part	Approach	Device	Qualifier
0 Head **1** Facial Muscle **2** Neck Muscle, Right **3** Neck Muscle, Left **4** Tongue, Palate, Pharynx Muscle **5** Shoulder Muscle, Right **6** Shoulder Muscle, Left **7** Upper Arm Muscle, Right **8** Upper Arm Muscle, Left **9** Lower Arm and Wrist Muscle, Right **B** Lower Arm and Wrist Muscle, Left **C** Hand Muscle, Right **D** Hand Muscle, Left **F** Trunk Muscle, Right **G** Trunk Muscle, Left **H** Thorax Muscle, Right **J** Thorax Muscle, Left **M** Perineum Muscle **N** Hip Muscle, Right **P** Hip Muscle, Left **Q** Upper Leg Muscle, Right **R** Upper Leg Muscle, Left **S** Lower Leg Muscle, Right **T** Lower Leg Muscle, Left **V** Foot Muscle, Right **W** Foot Muscle, Left	**0** Open **4** Percutaneous Endoscopic	**Z** No Device	**0** Skin **1** Subcutaneous Tissue **2** Skin and Subcutaneous Tissue **Z** No Qualifier
K Abdomen Muscle, Right **L** Abdomen Muscle, Left	**0** Open **4** Percutaneous Endoscopic	**Z** No Device	**0** Skin **1** Subcutaneous Tissue **2** Skin and Subcutaneous Tissue **6** Transverse Rectus Abdominis Myocutaneous Flap **Z** No Qualifier

Source: Adapted from ICD-10 Procedure Coding System (ICD-10-PCS) 2011 Tables and Index.

Access the ICD-10 Procedure Coding System (ICD-10-PCS) 2011 Tables and Index at www.cms.gov/ICD10/11b_2011_ICD10PCS.asp#TopOfPage.

Select 2011 Code Tables and Index.

Case Study 13

Correct answer:

0US94ZZ

Rationale:

For laparoscopic uterine suspension, the ICD-10-PCS Index references the first four characters of the 0US root operation table:

Suspension

Uterus *see* Reposition, Uterus 0US9

A review of the 0US root operation table and the operative report provides the information needed to assign the remaining three characters of the code:

Section:	0	Medical and surgical
Body system:	U	Female reproductive system
Operation:	S	Reposition: moving to its normal location, or other suitable location, all or a portion of a body part
Body part:	9	Uterus
Approach:	4	Percutaneous endoscopic
Device:	Z	No device
Qualifier:	Z	No qualifier

FIGURE 4.23

0US

Section	0	Medical and Surgical
Body System	U	Female Reproductive System
Operation	S	Reposition: Moving to its normal location or other suitable location all or a portion of a body part

Body Part	Approach	Device	Qualifier
0 Ovary, Right **1** Ovary, Left **2** Ovaries, Bilateral **4** Uterine Supporting Structure **5** Fallopian Tube, Right **6** Fallopian Tube, Left **7** Fallopian Tube, Bilateral **C** Cervix **F** Cul-de-sac	**0** Open **4** Percutaneous Endoscopic	**Z** No Device	**Z** No Qualifier
9 Uterus **G** Vagina	**0** Open **4** Percutaneous Endoscopic **X** External	**Z** No Device	**Z** No Qualifier

Source: Adapted from ICD-10 Procedure Coding System (ICD-10-PCS) 2011 Tables and Index.

Access the ICD-10 Procedure Coding System (ICD-10-PCS) 2011 Tables and Index at www.cms.gov/ICD10/11b_2011_ICD10PCS.asp#TopOfPage.

Select 2011 Code Tables and Index.

Case Study 14

Correct answer:

    0NH00NZ

    0NH00NZ

Rationale:

ICD-10-PCS Coding Guidelines 2011, guideline B4.3, states:

> Bilateral body part values are available for a limited number of body parts. If the identical procedure is performed on contralateral body parts, and a bilateral body part value exists for that body part, a single procedure is coded using the bilateral body part value. If no bilateral body part value exists, each procedure is coded separately using the appropriate body part value.

The ICD-10-PCS Index references all seven characters of the 0NH root operation table for placement of bilateral brain neurostimulator generators:

Neurostimulator Generator

    Insertion of device in, Skull 0NH00NZ

A review of the 0NH root operation table and the operative report provides the information needed to verify the code:

Section:	0	Medical and surgical
Body system:	N	Head and facial bones
Operation:	H	Insertion: putting in a nonbiological appliance that monitors, assists, performs, or prevents a physiological function but does not physically take the place of a body part
Body part:	0	Skull
Approach:	0	Open
Device:	N	Neurostimulator generator
Qualifier:	Z	No qualifier

FIGURE 4.24

0NH

Section	0	Medical and Surgical
Body System	N	Head and Facial Bones
Operation	H	Insertion: Putting in a nonbiological appliance that monitors, assists, performs, or prevents a physiological function but does not physically take the place of a body part

Body Part	Approach	Device	Qualifier
0 Skull	**0** Open	**4** Internal Fixation Device **5** External Fixation Device **M** Bone Growth Stimulator **N** Neurostimulator Generator	**Z** No Qualifier
0 Skull	**3** Percutaneous **4** Percutaneous Endoscopic	**4** Internal Fixation Device **5** External Fixation Device **M** Bone Growth Stimulator	**Z** No Qualifier
1 Frontal Bone, Right **2** Frontal Bone, Left **3** Parietal Bone, Right **4** Parietal Bone, Left **7** Occipital Bone, Right **8** Occipital Bone, Left **C** Sphenoid Bone, Right **D** Sphenoid Bone, Left **F** Ethmoid Bone, Right **G** Ethmoid Bone, Left **H** Lacrimal Bone, Right **J** Lacrimal Bone, Left **K** Palatine Bone, Right **L** Palatine Bone, Left **M** Zygomatic Bone, Right **N** Zygomatic Bone, Left **P** Orbital Bone, Right **Q** Orbital Bone, Left **X** Hyoid Bone	**0** Open **3** Percutaneous **4** Percutaneous Endoscopic	**4** Internal Fixation Device	**Z** No Qualifier
5 Temporal Bone, Right **6** Temporal Bone, Left	**0** Open **3** Percutaneous **4** Percutaneous Endoscopic	**4** Internal Fixation Device **S** Hearing Device	**Z** No Qualifier
B Nasal Bone	**0** Open **3** Percutaneous **4** Percutaneous Endoscopic	**4** Internal Fixation Device **M** Bone Growth Stimulator	**Z** No Qualifier

FIGURE 4.24		0NH (cont.)	

Body Part	Approach	Device	Qualifier
R Maxilla, Right **S** Maxilla, Left **T** Mandible, Right **V** Mandible, Left	**0** Open **3** Percutaneous **4** Percutaneous Endoscopic	**4** Internal Fixation Device **5** External Fixation Device	**Z** No Qualifier
W Facial Bone	**0** Open **3** Percutaneous **4** Percutaneous Endoscopic	**M** Bone Growth Stimulator	**Z** No Qualifier

Source: Adapted from ICD-10 Procedure Coding System (ICD-10-PCS) 2011 Tables and Index.

Access the ICD-10 Procedure Coding System (ICD-10-PCS) 2011 Tables and Index at www.cms.gov/ICD10/11b_2011_ICD10PCS.asp#TopOfPage.

Select 2011 Code Tables and Index.

Case Study 15

Correct answer:

0RRU0JZ

0RRU0JZ

0RRU0JZ

0RRU0JZ

Rationale:

Four codes are needed because the arthroplasty was performed on four MP joints.

ICD-10-PCS Coding Guidelines 2011, guideline B3.2, states:

> *During the same operative episode, multiple procedures are coded if: … The same root operation is repeated at different body sites that are included in the same body part value.*

A review of the 0RR root operation table and the operative report provides the information needed to verify the code:

Arthroplasty

see Replacement, Upper Joints 0RR

Section:	0	Medical and surgical
Body system:	R	Upper joints
Operation:	R	Replacement: putting in or on biological or synthetic material that physically takes the place and/or function of all or a portion of a body part
Body part:	U	Metacarpophalangeal joint, right
Approach:	0	Open
Device:	J	Synthetic substitute (Swanson implants)
Qualifier:	Z	No qualifier

FIGURE 4.25

0RR

Section	0	Medical and Surgical
Body System	R	Upper Joints
Operation	R	Replacement: Putting in a nonbiological appliance that monitors, assists, performs, or prevents a physiological function but does not physically take the place of a body part

Body Part	Approach	Device	Qualifier
0 Occipital-cervical Joint **1** Cervical Vertebral Joint **4** Cervicothoracic Vertebral Joint **6** Thoracic Vertebral Joint **A** Thoracolumbar Vertebral Joint	**0** Open	**7** Autologous Tissue Substitute **K** Nonautologous Tissue Substitute	**Z** No Qualifier
0 Occipital-cervical Joint **1** Cervical Vertebral Joint **4** Cervicothoracic Vertebral Joint **6** Thoracic Vertebral Joint **A** Thoracolumbar Vertebral Joint	**0** Open	**J** Synthetic Substitute	**4** Facet **Z** No Qualifier

---

FIGURE 4.25

0RR (cont.)

Body Part	Approach	Device	Qualifier
3 Cervical Vertebral Disc **5** Cervicothoracic Vertebral Disc **9** Thoracic Vertebral Disc **B** Thoracolumbar Vertebral Disc **C** Temporomandibular Joint, Right **D** Temporomandibular Joint, Left **E** Sternoclavicular Joint, Right **F** Sternoclavicular Joint, Left **G** Acromioclavicular Joint, Right **H** Acromioclavicular Joint, Left **L** Elbow Joint, Right **M** Elbow Joint, Left **N** Wrist Joint, Right **P** Wrist Joint, Left **Q** Carpal Joint, Right **R** Carpal Joint, Left **S** Metacarpocarpal Joint, Right **T** Metacarpocarpal Joint, Left **U** Metacarpophalangeal Joint, Right **V** Metacarpophalangeal Joint, Left **W** Finger Phalangeal Joint, Right **W** Finger Phalangeal Joint, Left	**0** Open	**7** Autologous Tissue Substitute **J** Synthetic Substitute **K** Nonautologous Tissue Substitute	**Z** No Qualifier
J Shoulder Joint, Right **K** Shoulder Joint, Left	**0** Open	**7** Autologous Tissue Substitute **K** Nonautologous Tissue Substitute	**Z** No Qualifier
J Shoulder Joint, Right **K** Shoulder Joint, Left	**0** Open	**J** Synthetic Substitute	**5** Reverse Ball and Socket **6** Humeral Surface **7** Glenoid Surface **Z** No Qualifier

Source: Adapted from ICD-10 Procedure Coding System (ICD-10-PCS) 2011 Tables and Index.

Access the ICD-10 Procedure Coding System (ICD-10-PCS) 2011 Tables and Index at www.cms.gov/ICD10/11b_2011_ICD10PCS.asp#TopOfPage.

Select 2011 Code Tables and Index.